Understanding Neuromuscular Plasticity

A basis for clinical rehabilitation

Geoffrey Kidd MSc, PhD
Director, Seminar College, Chester

Nigel Lawes MB, BS
Lecturer, Department of Biomedical Science,
University of Sheffield

and

Iris Musa PhD, MPhil, MSCP
Senior Lecturer, Cardiff School of Physiotherapy

Edward Arnold
A division of Hodder & Stoughton
LONDON   MELBOURNE   AUCKLAND

© 1992 Geoffrey Kidd, Nigel Lawes and Iris Musa

First published in Great Britain 1992

British Library Cataloguing in Publication Data

Kidd, Geoffrey MSc
  Understanding neuromuscular plasticity.
  I. Title II. Musa, Iris M. PhD
  III. Lawes, Nigel
  616.8

  ISBN 0-340-55244-1

Whilst the advice and information in this book is believed to be true
and accurate at the date of going to press, neither the author nor the
publisher can accept any legal responsibility or liability for any
errors or omissions that may be made. In particular (but without
limiting the generality of the preceding disclaimer) every effort has
been made to check drug dosages; however, it is still possible that
errors have been missed. Furthermore, dosage schedules are
constantly being revised and new side effects recognised. For these
reasons the reader is strongly urged to consult the drug companies'
printed instructions before administering any of the drugs
recommended in this book.

Typeset in 10/11pt Baskerville by Rowland Phototypesetting
Limited, Bury St Edmunds, Suffolk.
Printed and bound in Great Britain for Edward Arnold, a division
of Hodder and Stoughton Limited, Mill Road, Dunton Green,
Sevenoaks, Kent TN13 2YA by Butler and Tanner Limited, Frome
and London

Understanding Neuromuscular Plasticity

Contents

Foreword

Imagine a central nervous system you can mould and change through your hands. Imagine a spinal cord you can talk to and indeed converse with. Imagine being able to gain recovery of function after neurological or neuromuscular insult. Now stop imagining and enter a new world. In this excellent book you can read about the reality of the plasticity of the central nervous system. The central nervous system has the ability to adapt and change in response to input and environmental stimuli. The direction this takes can be either positive or negative, and its direction can most definitely be controlled by therapy.

So exciting, much more exciting than promoting compensation, adaptation and indeed the establishment of a new state. This is the reality of regaining normality as opposed to acquiring abnormality, eg., spastic hemiplegia.

The early part of the book explores both molecular and cellular neurobiology. It starts to establish the fundamental idea of **form function** as opposed to the old idea of **form** being separate from **function**. This idea is forward thinking.

Cyclical control means that by changing function in therapy one can change and adapt cell anatomy and physiology and vice versa. This means that therapy becomes a skilful, learning and purposeful experience. Anyone can make a hemiplegic patient walk with a tripod or use only one leg when rising from sitting to standing, but only a therapist with understanding and skill in directing neuroplasticity will bring about a positive recovery. These ideas are being explored daily by skilled therapists who so far have been unable to explain the results scientifically to physicians and neurologists.

This book will help to give both the medical and paramedical profession the ability to speak to each other in the same language for the benefit of the patient.

The central core of the book looks at the central nervous system in terms of flexible, adaptable, interacting components or systems rather than fixed stereotyped tracts of information. It is so refreshing to lose the old stereotyped mould and to open up one's mind towards creativity rather than compensation.

Finally we conclude with a review of therapy itself, which relays a very clear message: that effective therapeutic intervention needs to emphasize the facilitation of normal movement and to stress the central nervous system to learn.

Music to our ears.

Mary Lynch MSCP
Senior Tutor, Bobath Centre, London

Introduction

Life is an improbable state and the life of man is the most improbable state of all

Young, 1947

The intention is to write a book which presents a picture of the nervous system that is alive. A nervous system that is so specifically alive as to be able to adapt to changes forced upon it during development and during recovery from disease and injury. A nervous system sufficiently complex to control human behaviour and sufficiently flexible in its complexity to restore human behaviour once it has been impaired.

The contents list indicates clearly the priorities that have been adopted. Plasticity must be defined before any discussion can be started. The widely held view that regeneration in the human central nervous system is not yet practicable does not mean it never will be so. Failure to understand plastic adaptation will delay its application by the widely ranging techniques of clinical rehabilitation. A realistic definition to which we will return, time and time again as the book progresses, is given by Brown and Hardman (1987):

> ... the ability of cells to alter any aspect of their phenotype, at any stage in development, in response to abnormal changes in their state or environment.

There will be no analysis of the holistic philosophy of nervous action. Instead, there will be a synthesis that will lead towards an understanding of that critical interaction of neurons which allows a wonderful weave from the warp and the weft of individual neural responses called action currents.

An introduction to those macromolecules which are sufficiently complex to act as molecular machines is presented. This takes us into the concept that aggregates of molecules are able to act as components of the cells which comprise the neuromuscular systems. Starting in this way, from the molecule, can up-end conventional concepts and also unbalance the usually seen divisions of the academic disciplines (Fig. 1). Discussion of the cell

FORM	FUNCTION
Anatomy	Physiology
Neuroanatomy	Neurophysiology
Histology : Cytology	Cell physiology

Bioch *em* istry

See the anatomy of the biochemistry doing the physiology

Fig. 1 The early disciplines concentrating on form and function, i.e. anatomy and physiology, specialized and became more relevant to clinical rehabilitation. The two lines of specialization united into a bioch *em* istry of macromolecules which in the *e*lectron *m*icroscope allowed us to visualize the anatomy of the biochemistry doing the physiology.

nucleus will follow later. The nuclei will be presented as controllers of the cells which, in response to significant changes in cellular or organism environment, allow expression of the genes they contain. Such activity forms the basis of cellular neurobiology and its application to a study of neuromuscular plasticity. Neurobiology is defined, and beautifully expounded, by Shepherd (1988):

> Neurobiology is the study of the molecular organization of the nerve cell, and the ways that nerve cells are organized, through synapses, into functional circuits that process information and mediate behaviour.

Chapter 1 An introduction to neurobiology

Neuroscience, when it is appropriate to the subject being presented, admits to the discussion of measurements with the dimensions of linear and solid geometry, of time and of concentration, and the way in which those parameters change with time. Time itself requires unusual descriptions (Fig. 2).

Chronological time has only one dimension and is limited in value unless it is used to explain how some other parameter is changing with respect to it. Psychological time again has a limited value. It

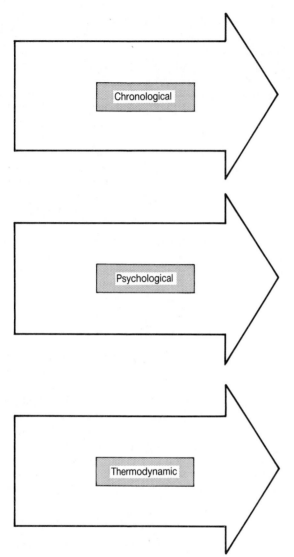

Fig. 2 We must be comfortable with three time scales. The first is the one usually considered, and we believe, considered too much. The processes of rehabilitation do not fit easily into chronological time. Similarly, psychological time which deals with our past and our future is distorting. It is thermodynamic time which is concerned with the changing probabilities of molecules being present in the neuromuscular system which guides us to the correct understanding of plastic adaptation.

tells us what was in the past, allows us to define the present and lets us anticipate the future.

Thermodynamic time measures the amount of change there is in the order or disorder (the entropy) of a system. The total entropy of a non-

living system is forever tending towards a maximum, corresponding to complete disorder. A growing, remembering and rehabilitating living system exhibits negative entropy (negentropy): a state in which order is increasing.

Chapter 2   An introduction to cellular neurobiology

This chapter can be thought of as the mirror image of Chapter 1. Presented there are examples of how molecules and molecular systems can increase in complexity and interaction until they can show just how the cells are composed and able to manifest the properties of an irritability which leads to an excitation, and indeed to the responses characteristic of life itself. Here, the analysis is in the terms of neurobiology, the fine details of cell morphology until it defies further expression in any way other than in molecular terms. The large number of varieties of neurons in the brain will be simplified in an ordered way so that the mind is not bewildered by numbers of astronomical dimension.

The techniques of histology will be presented not to impress you with types of neuron available to our study, but in a way that leads us to learn the essential simplicity of the diverse neuronal forms, and the richness that molecular mutability brings to the subject of neuronal plastic adaptation.

Chapter 3   Transmission of signals by neurons

The action potential of an excitable cell, for example, a neuron or a muscle fibre (although strictly speaking a muscle fibre is a syncitium in which primitive muscle cells, myoblasts, have fused end-to-end during development) is a cyclic change of state and lasts for a time of the order of 1.0 and 10.0 milliseconds (1.0–10.0 ms). It is sometimes described as being all-or-nothing in character. The amplitude of the potential, but not of the magnitude of current flowing as a consequence of excitation, is a factor of membrane characteristic and not of stimulus intensity.

More exactly, it is a phenomenon determined by the cell membrane and the changing concentration of ions in the extracellular and intracellular fluid phases it separates. An action potential cannot be said to be conducted. In an excitable cell such as a neuron, an action potential is generated by a patch of membrane. It is generated there, it decays there and the currents that its generates in the conducting extracellular and intracellular fluids give rise to a new action potential in the nearest, and usually the most excitable, adjacent patch of membrane.

The disciplines of neurobiology and neuroscience can be very dry. They come alive only as they offer an explanation of the dynamics of a nervous system adapting to meet the need for change: change as in growth or as in recovery after injury and disablement.

By this stage, the book will have introduced to you the complexity of the macromolecules of excitable cells and you will have an insight into the probability of their existence. The improbability associated with the complexity of living structures leads to some instability and to an impermanence and readiness to change. This changeability is predictable and controllable and leads to an effective clinical rehabilitation of the neuromuscular system.

Chapter 4 Synaptic transmission

There is a mutability of macromolecules, both of their form and of their location within neurons and muscle fibres. This allows the operation of plastic adaptation of the neuromuscular system. The adaptive process is however too slow, during the short term, to act in regulations required for the control of an ongoing movement.

The all-or-nothing characteristic (see Chapter 3) of action potentials distinguishes between threshold and subthreshold changes in neuron excitability and between threshold and subthreshold stimuli. The development of local, graded and non-propagated potentials (and also the associated current flows) across cell membranes occurs at synapses between neurons and synapses between neurons and muscle fibres.

It is at the neuronal synapses that an element of uncertainty of response is introduced into the central nervous system. The all-or-nothing nature of the action potential is replaced by a dual control of the amplitude of membrane potential change. The release of neurotransmitter by the action currents generated by the potential entering the synapse releases molecules of a neurotransmitter from the presynapic membrane which reacts with receptor molecules in the postsynaptic membrane.

Information is contained in the effect of reaction between molecules of neurotransmitter and the receptor molecules to which they bind. Information is transmitted about the importance which must be attached to an action current with respect to discharge of an action potential in the postsynaptic neuron in the chain. Synaptic effects are able to add together (summate). A single synaptic effect is seldom able by itself to cause discharge of the next neuron. Indeed, the subthreshold excitatory and inhibitory effects exert an important element of control. This is through a form of algebraic summation in which inhibition can disturb the balance of, or indeed cancel, an excitatory action. The process of inhibition and excitation are customarily abbreviated to −ve and +ve, respectively.

The changing activity of transmitter molecules and receptor molecules, during the procedure of plastic adaptation, can be brought about intentionally with the techniques of clinical rehabilitation. A description of how this can be done is the major purpose of this book.

Chapter 5 Plasticity in development and redevelopment

To live is to change and to be perfect is to have changed often.

John Henry Newman

There are some ten billion nerve cells in the brain, each of which makes about ten thousand contacts with other nerve cells – one hundred trillion connections in all. Yet despite these unimaginably large numbers, these connections are highly ordered. Every square millimetre of skin, for example, is innervated by nerve fibres that project to precise areas in the sensory cortex in such an ordered way that a map of the body can be drawn on the cortex. The connections are so highly ordered, in fact, that there are not enough genes to code for them all. There are also a large number of different types of neuron in the brain, each of which can be found in specific locations. Each neuron has characteristic patterns of dendritic and axonal trees; each makes predictable connections with other neurons. If this represents too much order, or information, for the entire genome to contain, how do the cells 'know' what to become, which dendritic trees to grow, which molecules of transmitter to synthesize, which connections to make?

Every cell in the body contains the genetic information necessary to become every other cell. Cells in the nose contain the genes for cells in the toes for example. Most genes have to be switched off, so that toes do not sprout on noses, but the relevant genes also have to be switched on (expressed). This chapter will outline some of what is known about how a neuron finds out what to become and what connections to make during development. It will be shown that every neuronal modification is the result of local environmental clues turning genes on and off, so that development is a plastic process, varying with local condition. The interaction between extracellular cues and intracellular genes specifies neuron type, neuron location and neuron connections during the process of development. It will be argued that although these developmental interactions occur at a given time, called a critical period, and are then switched off, they can be reactivated when required. Reactivation of plastic processes is instigated whenever the local environment changes significantly. A change in the use of a limb or the stimulation to which it is exposed will, for instance, change its cerebro-cortical representation, the dendritic trees of the neurons connected to it, and even the connections of these neurons to each other. Similar changes occur after injury. It will be argued that learning and the responses to injury both utilize interactions between a neuron's environment and its genes similar to those that led to its development in the first place. This chapter will outline the phenomenology of development, learning and response to injury.

Chapter 6   Review of the control of movement as a component of 'classical' clinical neurophysiology

This chapter will look at the control of movement as a component of 'classical' neurophysiology. It will address the following question: Why do we need to look at 'classical' neurophysiology in an exposition on the plasticity of the neuromuscular system?

The quotation which opens this synopsis is appropriate in that the neuromuscular system develops and changes due to the activity of the individual and in order to adapt to the environment. Once it has reached maturity it does not become static but continues to change in response to the environment, particularly after damage. How the environment shapes the neuromuscular system is important if we are to understand how we can help to influence the shaping. How the environment continues to shape the system during maturity, through the effects of afferent input to the central nervous system (CNS) is important also

as these forces come into their own following damage to the CNS. These forces can be guided and assisted.

The classical stimulus–response physiology is still needed: it exists, and we need it, in the knowledge of its long-term effects in shaping and reshaping the neuromuscular system. In the natural environment, stimulus–response is accompanied by a trophic effect which changes or reinforces the response for the future. Applied artificially a stimulus–response approach may not contain this *trophic code*. The *code* must be identified if artificial stimulation is to be used. However, naturally occurring stimuli can be manipulated in order to achieve and reinforce not only the stimulus–response in therapy, but also the trophic effect. Stimulus–response must first be described as it is known in relation to movement control before it can be manipulated to the benefit, for example, of the brain-damaged patient.

This chapter will discuss therefore the development of the nervous system control of movement. It will look at the role of the spinal cord in movement control and also at the effects of activity, descending from the brain, and coming from the periphery onto the spinal cord. A study of the role of afferent input from the periphery on the CNS control of movement is of particular importance if we are to understand how we can manipulate afferent input in order to best guide the nervous system in its adaptation to a changing environment.

Chapter 7   The plasticity of skeletal muscle: its direction by training effects and by electrotherapy

This chapter will introduce the response of skeletal muscle (striated muscle) to changes which bring about an adaptive response better to meet the requirements of human motor performance.

Skeletal muscle is under the control of alpha-motoneurons (skeleto-motoneurons). Consequently, this chapter will be presented in such a way that the development and maintenance of the neuromuscular system will show clearly their interdependence. This interdependence will emphasize the need for contact between nerve and muscle, and for matching of muscle characteristics with the discharge pattern of motoneuron activity.

Particular attention will be given to the neuromuscular junction and the presence and distribution of acetylcholine (ACh) receptors during early development, and to the stability of the interdependence during the maintenance of maturity. A recapitulation of some of the stages of early development will be provided and examined during the procedures of clinical rehabilitation which follows some injuries of the neuromuscular system.

A future projection of an applicable neurophysiology will be made as an expansion of the definition by Sherrington (1904) of the muscle unit of the motor unit as 'the final common path of the motor system'. That it is a 'final common path' which has been taken into the thinking of neurophysiology, almost by osmosis. We must not think, in these later days, that the definition is fully adequate. If it were so, clinical rehabilitation would not be possible. Bernard Shaw's apothegm 'Doctors keep the patient amused, whilst nature effects the cure' should be modified to '. . . whilst plastic adaptation takes effect'.

What will be treated here is the detail of the mechanisms of skeletal muscle adaption to meet functional requirements. This almost encyclopaedic subject will cover the responses to different forms of activity during habilation (a form of physical education whereby the normal adaptation of the neuromuscular system from neonate to maturity is encouraged, pursued or prescribed). Rehabilitation is a carefully planned and directed return to the processes of habilation once, as a consequence of insult or accident, they have been impaired or temporarily lost. The main arguments of early thoughts on habilation and rehabilitation will form the subject matter of chapters 6 and 9, respectively.

The theoretical basis of clinical rehabilitation has by now progressed so far that it is feasible to construct a therapy designed specifically to direct and guide plastic adaptation. These contemporary techniques need the establishment of insights by you, and the application of mind, again by you the readers (never confuse the application of mind with remembering: the first is active and, more often than not, the second is passive).

In essence, the contemporary techniques of clinical rehabilitation consist of deciphering the codes used by the CNS as it conveys information to damaged centres within itself and conveys it also to damaged or diseased skeletal muscle. Information is transmitted through the neuromuscular system by a series of linked modifications of molecules and it is this that is required to bring about an appropriate and necessary adaptation.

Electrotherapies, notably *eutrophic* electrotherapies (the adjective *eutrophic* qualifies an electrotherapy which has been calculated ideally to produce an optimal trophic effect on the cells being involved in adaptation) which introduces, at first as a copy or approximation of the code and latterly as a code calculated exactly, instructions to the cells on the direction in which adaptation of the tissue is to proceed. In this manner, existing electrotherapies were improved upon and previously unthought of therapies enabled.

Chapter 8 The mechanisms of development and redevelopment

When the expression 'synaptic strength' is used accurately (for a fine example of this refer to Kandel, 1981) it embodies almost the whole topic of plastic adaptation of the CNS. Linking such diverse phenomena as simple potentiation and memory, synaptic strengthening becomes very much a 'short-hand' ideogram. It is, though, too important a concept in the understanding of neuroscience as a basis of clinical rehabilitation to remain just that.

Four types of synaptic plasticity contributing to synaptic strength can be distinguished:

1. Post-tetanic potentiation
2. Low-frequency depression

Types 1 and 2 are homosynaptic in their plastic adaptation (the reader should be remedying unfamiliarity with some of the words used here by referring to the Glossary in the Appendix to this book).

The complement of four types of synaptic plasticity is completed by:

3. Heterosynaptic plasticity of excitatory synapses
4. Heterosynaptic plasticity of inhibitory synapses

The significance of this latter plastic adaptation is discussed in Chapter 9.

Once again, the present chapter concentrates the attention on those molecules and their form and position within the neuronal membrane which contains the presynaptic and postsynaptic macromolecular arrays.

The main points of Chapter 4 will be reintroduced here with the objective of making the reader more comfortable with an approach to clinical rehabilitation based mainly on the properties of macromolecules. It is the mutability of such molecules which allows the fusion of the characteristics of FORM and FUNCTION into the concept of FORMFUNCTION. Without this, an understanding of the possible techniques of clinical rehabilitation would be difficult to apply.

Imagine synaptic strengthening developing in response to a coherent form of therapy. The response reproduces, throughout that particular form of time (thermodynamic time), a negentropy which develops usefully. The circuits of the CNS undergo a type of synaptic strengthening which links neurons into 'sets', each one of which is able to operate as a preferred element. Habilitation operates by means of set formation, and rehabilitation does also. It is an inevitable consequence of specifically applied therapies.

In Chapter 5, observations on how nerve cells behave during development, learning and regeneration were given. In this chapter, the cellular and molecular mechanisms underlying these phenomena will be explored. Some of the differences between axons and dendrites will be sketched, including differential axonal transport (see also Chapter 3, section 3.2, p. 34). The neuritic growth cone, central to the whole development and redevelopment of the nervous system, will be described, together with some of the factors which govern its behaviour. Glutamate receptor subtypes will be described to illustrate how learning takes place at a cellular level. The roles of calcium (see also Chapter 1), calmodulin, kinases, GAP43 and other relevant ions and molecules will be alluded to. Once the molecular mechanisms of learning have been laid down, evidence showing that the same mechanisms are involved in development and in regeneration will be given, tying together all three phenomena.

Chapter 9   A critical review of contemporary therapies

This chapter will present a brief history of therapeutic approaches to rehabilitation of CNS dysfunction and a critique of contemporary therapies. The critique will be based on the ability of the therapies to guide plastic adaptation in the CNS in order to achieve, restore or maintain normal movement and function in the long-term.

The therapies need to be able to:

1. Strengthen normal synaptic chains and neuronal sets.

2. Guide axonal sprouting.
3. Facilitate the unmasking of alternative or previously subservient pathways in the CNS in order to maintain normal function through alternative routes.

To return to 'classical' stimulus–response physiology: in the short-term, what goes in determines what comes out. However, the ability of the CNS to adapt plastically means, in the longer term, that what goes in modifies the inside so that it can more easily give the same response in the future. So abnormal movements in the short-term will reinforce abnormal movements in the long-term by making it easier for the CNS to respond to the same stimulus in the future. In the main, therapies are based on stimulus–response but if the response is abnormal it will be reinforced. A knowledge of stimulus–response is necessary in order to appreciate the basis for therapies, but a knowledge of plastic adaptation alters our understanding of their effect and therefore determines their future development. The development and treatment of spasticity can serve as an example of plastic adaptation within the CNS but handling techniques may be able to guide the adaptation (particularly heterosynaptic plastic adaptation of inhibitory synapses) to make it more normal and therefore improve function in the long-term. Arguments for the causes of spasticity and for approaches to its management and treatment will be presented. The chapter will look at the following contemporary approaches:

1. Neurodevelopmental approaches
2. Proprioceptive neuromuscular facilitation
3. The Bobath approach
4. Conductive education
5. Doman–Delacato method

The chapter will conclude with a suggested blueprint for effective therapeutic intervention based on the arguments presented throughout the book.

References

Brown, M. C. and Hardman, V. J. (1987). Plasticity of vertebrate motoneurons. In: Winlow, W. and McCrohan, C. R. (1987) *Growth and Plasticity of Nerve Connection*. University Press, Manchester.

Sherrington, C. S. (1904). *The correlation of reflexes and the principle of the common final path*. British Association, **74**: 727-741.

Young, J. Z. (1974). *The Introduction to the Study of Man*. Cambridge Univerity Press, Cambridge.

Chapter 1

An introduction to molecular neurobiology

> It is not art that rains down upon us in the song of a bird; but the simplest modulation, correctly executed is already art.
>
> Poetics of Music, Igor Stravinski

Molecular neurobiology is a vast subject, becoming even more vast as we write. There is no intention here of exhausting its contents. It will take all the space we can allow to introduce you to the molecules of the neuron and muscle fibre and give you a sense of the restlessness of molecular interaction which represents the dynamic of plastic adaptation of the neuromuscular system.

1.1 Body water

> Water, water everywhere and yet no drop to drink
> Water, water everywhere and still the molecules shrink
>
> with apologies to Coleridge

The scientific basis of rehabilitation requires an introduction to molecular biology. We have no intention of baffling you but we must move away from the attitudes exaggerated somewhat by Fig. 1.1a.

The hands are most certainly marvellous, and the movement required can be demonstrated time and time again. You should realize however, that the black box contains not only the whole of the neuromuscular system and the cells which comprise it, but additionally the molecules from which the cells themselves are assembled. The mutability of those molecules gives rise to the plastic adaptation as it is initiated and controlled by the therapist.

To press the subject of the black box too hard is almost an insult to your profession, so to redress the insult we should consider Fig. 1.1b. Combine the exaggerations of both Figs 1.1a and b and something like the truth emerges. Let us drill a few holes into the black box and allow the fresh air of a different philosophy to enter.

We will describe some molecular assemblies in an example of one of the constructive ways of rearranging your thoughts. The most complex molecules from which we are constructed were themselves assembled or synthesized in water. Figure 1.2 illustrates the distribution of body water. Total body water is contained in three compartments: 1 is the compartment inside the cells and is described as being intracellular, compartment 2 is contained in the interstices between cells and is called interstitial for that reason, whereas 3 is the water component of blood plasma which circulates around the other two as it refreshes and replenishes them.

We will return to the important subject of what it is that separates such things as individual action potentials in Chapter 8, Section 8.6, but we should introduce here the importance of the boundaries between the three compartments of body water. The total body water is a continuum, an uninterrupted phase of water into which is synthesized the molecules forming boundaries with differing permeabilities for the components of body fluid.

The membrane forming the boundary which separates the plasma and the interstitial fluid phases has the property of semipermeability. More

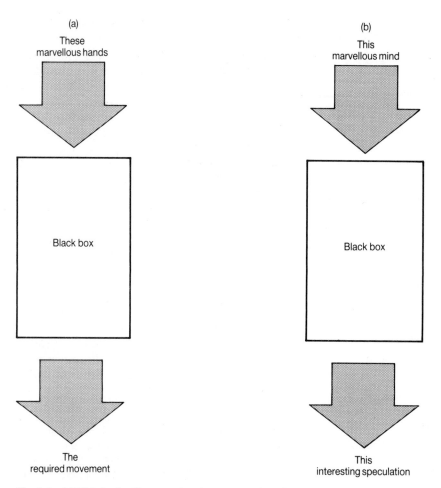

Fig. 1.1 (a) This book will re-examine the contents of the BLACK BOX which contains all of the neurons, the muscle fibres and the molecules from which they are formed. Your hands *are* marvellous and the required movements *are* obtained. (b) The exaggeration in (a) is intentional but it is balanced by the exaggeration here. A different look at the neuromuscular system is presented by this book.

simply, the membrane distinguishes only what it will allow to pass on the basis of molecular size. The plasma proteins, for example, are normally prevented from entering the interstitial fluid phase. This is because of their relatively large size and diameter. Small molecules of crystalloid compounds and gases can, by comparison, diffuse freely. It is the porous wall of the capillary network which gives it semipermeability.

The exchange of solutes (substances dissolved) between the interstitial and the intracellular fluid phases is controlled by the selective permeability of the plasma membranes which form the cell walls. In Chapter 3, Section 3.1, we will describe the molecular structure and the activity of some of the

ion pumps which contribute to the selectivity of transport.

The semipermeability and selective permeability of two of the membranes separating the body fluid compartments are illustrated by Fig. 1.3 where the shading of the three compartments follows that used for Fig. 1.2.

1.2 Structure of intracellular water of the neuromuscular system

The interaction between molecules of water and the substances dissolved in it confers a structure upon both of them that is an essential component of the adaptive plasticity of the neuromuscular

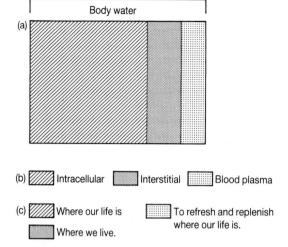

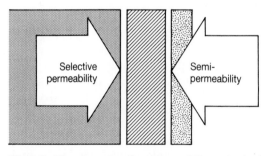

Fig. 1.2 The total body water is contained in compartments bounded by cell membranes. We should think more about where our life is. Where we live must also be considered. The water of the blood plasma assists in refreshing and replenishing the other two.

Fig. 1.3 The properties of semipermeability and selective permeability characterize the two living membranes which are the boundaries of the three compartments. An understanding of their structure will come from an understanding of the macromolecules of living membranes.

system. Water molecules, in the absence of any solute, form a tetrahedral lattice which has a structure with almost the precision of an ice crystal. This structure is illustrated in Fig. 1.4. The atoms of oxygen and hydrogen combine to form the molecule of water: H_2O. The chemical bonds which tie together the three atoms are known as covalent bonds. These bonds satisfy the laws of chemical combination and this bonding is shown along the bottom of the Fig, 1.4. In a small molecule such as water, the positive ($+ve$) electric charge on the two hydrogen atoms does not balance exactly the negative ($-ve$) electric charge on the oxygen atom and the resulting molecule is known as a dipole.

This point will be expanded in Chapter 3, Section 3.1. A second form of bonding between atoms further balances their electric charge by holding the molecules of water together by a lattice of hydrogen bonds (see Fig. 1.4).

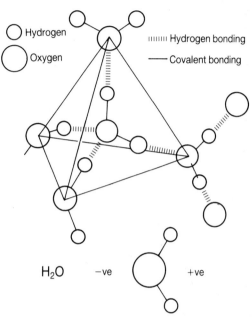

Fig. 1.4 In the absence of solutes, water can be thought of as a molecular lattice. The water molecule is a dipole (a structure charged electrically to be $+ve$ and $-ve$ at each end). Covalent bonds hold together the H_2O components. The tetrahedral structure is formed by hydrogen bonds which make use of the electric charge on the dipole.

This form of lattice work bonding holds some of the water molecules together in the tetrahedral form in all of the states between ice ($0°$ C) and when water as it is warmed absorbs enough energy in the form of heat to reach boiling point ($100°$ C). At that temperature, most of the hydrogen bonds are broken and the liquid vapourizes. In the intracellular phase at body temperature ($38°$ C) approximately 25% of the water of muscle fibres is in crystalline form (Dyson, 1974) as other intracellular molecules, notably protein molecules, reinforce the strength of the hydrogen bonds and hold the tetrahedral structure together.

Constraints on the arrangement of water molecules holding NaCl in solution is illustrated by Fig. 1.5 which shows the dipole form of the water molecule holding and being held by the electric charges of the Na^+ and the Cl^- ions (see also Chap-

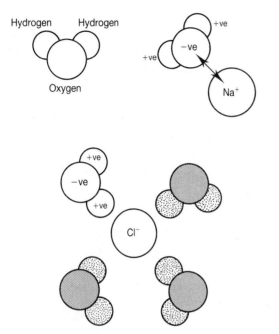

Fig. 1.5   The electric charge on the dipole forms a fluid anatomy with sodium and chloride ions (Na^+ and Cl^-). A hydrosphere of water molecules surrounds and protects the exposed ions of Na and Cl.

ter 3, Section 3.1 for a different approach to this point).

1.3   One, two, three, many . . . a form of counting used by Polynesian natives

The molecule from which proteins are formed is known as amino acid. When amino acids are linked the chemical bond that is formed is known as a peptide bond. The result of this bonding has various names. When a small number of amino acids are polymerized or bonded together the resulting molecule is known as an *oligopeptide*. When a polymer contains a larger number of amino acids it is referred to as a *polypeptide*.

A subtle difference starts to appear in a *polypeptide* molecule as the number of amino acids from which it is composed increases. The prefixes *oligo-* and *poly-* become almost meaningless and some other form of peptide classification is needed. The convention adopted is to qualify the form in which the peptide (*oligo-* or *poly-*) exists. If we were to discuss geometry in a similar way, we would employ, for example, the words: LINE, AREA and VOLUME.

Referring to Fig. 1.6, we could develop the geometric concept: LINE = the simplest or primary structure (abbreviated to 1^0) structure. Similarly, AREA = the secondary (2^0) and VOLUME = tertiary (3^0) structures as the concept becomes more revealing and more powerful in relation to this type of geometry.

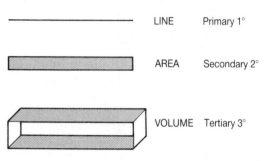

Fig. 1.6   The three simple geometric forms LINE, AREA and VOLUME are referred to as the primary (1^0), secondary (2^0) and tertiary (3^0) geometric structures. This diagram will help you to understand the three different structures of the protein molecule.

Returning to the subject of polypeptides, they can be described in a first approximation as having a 1^0 structure. Here, the polypeptide structure would be nothing more than a listed sequence of occurrence of the amino acids contained: ARGinine bonded to LEUcine which is bonded to PHEnylalanine followed by CYSteine and METhionine.

A description of the 2^0 structure would allow for the angle of the peptide bond between the individual amino acids (see Fig. 1.7).

Chemical characteristics of some amino acids, e.g. CYSteine can form bonds attractive to CYSteine elsewhere in the chain molecule, PROline as another example can act as a terminator amino acid in a polypeptide. Any S–S bond forming between two CYSteine molecules can cause folding in the polypeptide chain. Two forms of folding are possible: in one of them the molecule adopts a helical or coiled form and is called an alpha-helix. In the other a folded sheet form is adopted and is known as a beta-sheet. When the different forms can be described and their relationship with each other is defined an information-rich 3^0 structure is obtained. The polypeptide structure has not only increased in complexity, it has become a source of information which can be transferred within a cell and between different cells. It is a similar situation in concept development to the treatment by Ein-

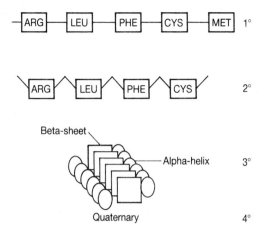

Fig. 1.7 A list of successive chemical names (i.e. of amino acids) gives us the simplest (1^0) structural formula of a protein. This represents LINE in Fig. 1.6. A more complex structural formula (2^0) takes into account the angle formed by the peptide bonds which link amino acids. A consideration of the structural complexity of polypeptide molecules in a protein gives the 3^0 form.

stein of the concepts of SPACE and TIME and the development of the more powerful concept of SPACETIME with its application to research into atomic structure and into the exploration of astronomical space (see Fig. 1.8). Further discussion of the 3^0 structure of polypeptides will be given in Chapter 3.

In Chapter 8 another concept of equivalent power to SPACETIME in the context of 3^0 structure of proteins will be introduced. FORMFUNCTION is used there in the description of plastic

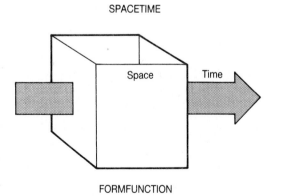

Fig. 1.8 The concept of SPACETIME developed by Einstein opened new forms of research into atomic structure and the exploration of space. A comparable but weaker concept of FORMFUNCTION is introduced to help research into neuromuscular plasticity.

adaptation of skeletal muscle: any modification of the FORM of skeletal muscle is followed by an alteration of its FUNCTION. Similarly, modifying the FUNCTION of a muscle results in a change in its FORM. Again it must be emphasized that this discussion is being carried out at a molecular level, and the topic is still molecular neurobiology.

A further order of structures has to be introduced, namely the quaternary (4^0) structure where the protein complex of polypeptides has associated molecular groupings or prosthetic groups. These operate in the neuromuscular system as conjugated proteins. The prosthetic group in conjugation with the polypeptide chains can be as simple as a metallic ion. In the molecule of myoglobin, the oxygen-carrying pigment of skeletal muscle, the protein globin is conjugated to Fe^{2+} carried by a porphyrin molecule. In the conjugated molecule of glycoprotein the complex carries a carbohydrate molecule. Glycoproteins form a component in the molecule of the membrane ion pumps discussed in Chapter 3, Section 3.1.

1.4 There are more things between heaven and earth, Horatio . . .

In addition to presenting an outstanding textbook, Shepherd (1988) uses a splendid turn of phrase. In drawing together what is common to all of neurobiology he refers to '*the biomolecular quartet*'. This has as players molecules called fatty acids, others which are called carbohydrates and take the form of simple sugars. You will realize already that amino acids join the *ensemble* that is completed by nucleic acids: the molecules which carry information in biological systems.

In one example, the molecular complexity that typifies the components of a *living* organism is formed by a process of *polymerization*. In simple organic chemistry a polymer is formed by the union of two or more molecules of the same compound to form larger molecules resulting in a new compound with the same empirical formula but of greater molecular weight. In another chemistry, called biochemistry, the appropriate complexity is formed when reactive groups at one end of the molecule bond to differing molecules. An example of this is shown in Fig. 1.9.

The elaboration of dipeptides and polypeptides of appropriate structural complexity to be called proteins has been discussed already. In general, this branch of organic chemistry treats a class of

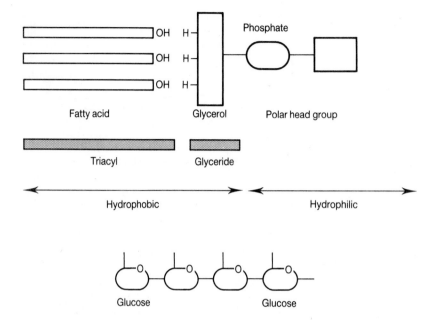

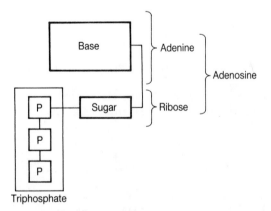

Fig. 1.9 The structure of a molecule, triacyl glyceride, from which fats can be formed is an attempt to introduce your minds to one way in which a molecule can be understood. The relationship of the molecule with body water is shown as 'water hating' and 'water liking' divisions of the molecule. A pictorial representation of another polymer, glycogen, is shown by a different diagram.

molecules called *monomers* and describes how two of them may react and become *dimers*. The elaboration of *polymers* from *monomers* and *dimers* completes the process.

The biomolecular quartet has a number of functional roles to play in the FORMFUNCTION of the neuromuscular system. As simple molecules, for example, glucose and amino acids, they serve as substrates for the enzymes involved in metabolism. In polymer form, glucose is stored in skeletal muscle fibres as glycogen where it acts as an energy reserve. Energy is also stored in the form of large molecules in depots throughout the body. In skeletal muscle fibres they are the triacyl glycerides (cf. Fig. 1.9) which act as a complementary energy reserve to glycogen.

A combination of basic molecular forms, i.e. as glycolipids and glycoproteins, serve as structural components of the cell membrane and as loci of molecular reception. Glycoprotein molecules are also able to act as an active component of the neuron membrane where they are able to operate as ion pumps (see Chapter 1, Section 1.6). The combination of molecular forms is important when they act as carriers of information within the cell. In this context, the information carried is used during molecular copying and during the synthesis of novel molecules. One of the information carriers is illustrated in Figs 1.10 and 1.11.

A combination of deoxyribose (a simple sugar) with either of the organic bases – purine or pyrimidine – and coupled to a phosphate group is known as a nucleotide. There is no intention to introduce more details of organic chemistry here. Reference to the Appendix will introduce more advanced detail for those who wish to understand better the structure of the molecules discussed. Polymerization of nucleotides yields nucleic acid, which polymerizes further to give deoxyribose nucleic acid: a molecule known better as DNA (Fig. 1.11).

Fig. 1.10 Another diagrammatic representation dissects the adenosine triphosphate (ATP) molecule. An organic base (adenine) is combined with a five-carbon sugar (a pentose called ribose) which carries three phosphate groups.

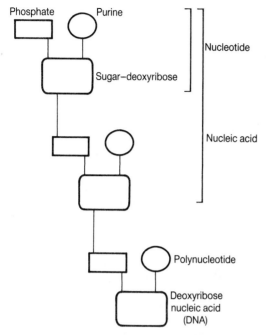

Fig. 1.11 A diagrammatic representation of the molecules which polymerize (see text) to form DNA. A nucleotide (the sugar deoxyribose combined with the base, purine, with a phosphate group) forms a dimer called nucleic acid. Polymerization of this acid forms a polynucleotide **d**eoxy**r**ibose **n**ucleic **a**cid.

1.5 STRESS as a change in environment

The straight run of the argument requires some redirecting, and before picking up conformity once again, it would be better to explore exactly what is the change in environment to which the neuromuscular system has to adapt.

The two factors of neuromuscular response to *a significant change in environment* is shown in Figs 1.12 a and b.

What was once called a *stimulus* is better referred to now as *a significant change in environment*. The main advantage of this is to encourage a partial break from a stimulus–response mode of thought. A *significant change in environment* does indeed have in it a component that we can still call a *stimulus*. But related inseparably to it is an element of *stress*, or more exactly a number of *stressors* which together act as a *stress* (see Fig. 1.12c).

For any significant change in environment the proportion of *stimulus* to *stress* need not be equal as in the manner in which it is shown in Fig. 1.12a.

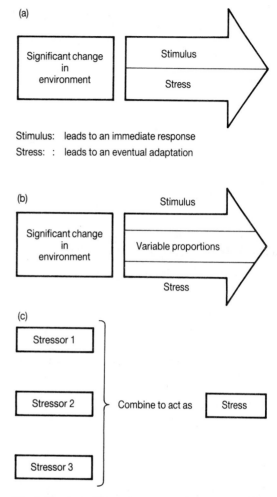

Stimulus: leads to an immediate response

Stress: : leads to an eventual adaptation

Fig. 1.12 A significant change in environment to which the neuromuscular system adapts. (a) The *stimulus* component leads to an immediate response of the system as the stimulus finds it. The *stress* component gives rise to an eventual adaptation of the system itself. (b) The proportion of stimulus to stress is variable. (c) A control of the degree of variability is the objective of the therapist. You should be recognizing by now the *stressors* which combine to act as a physiological stress and not be restricting yourselves to an application of stimulus alone.

The proportions of each are variable, and an achievement of an appropriate mix of *stimulus* and *stress* should be the objective of the therapist (Fig. 1.12b). Not all of this approach is either hypothetical or speculative. When therapists pay as much attention to *stressors* as they do to simple *stimuli* much will be learned by the neuroscientist to the mutual advantage of both professions.

The response of the neuromuscular system to

such a combination of *stress* and *stimulus* is shown in Fig. 1.12a as being firstly an immediate response of the system as the *stimulus* component finds it. The *stress* component leads to an eventual plastic adaptation. The duration of time taken to comply with the eventuality of the adaptation is employed by the cells of the nervous and muscular systems in becoming involved in molecular modification and replacement.

There must be a clear distinction in your minds between *stress* as a physiological variable and *stress* as a psychological one. Both usages are valid within their respective contexts. Here, we shall discuss *physiological* stressors and stress only.

1.6   Of ships and string and sealing wax, and molecules that move

The time when synaptic transmission depended only for its effectiveness on two or three simple neurotransmitter molecules is long past. The debates between opposing schools of thought on the 'spark or soup' modes of synaptic transmission (cf. Chapter 3, Section 3.2) has faded into fond memory. The so-called classical neurotransmitters, acetyl choline and adrenaline, still give us choliner-*gic* and adren*ergic* as classifiers which emphasize that the synaptic effectiveness is due to the name of the molecule prefixed. Accordingly, there is added to the neuropharmacological compendium needed for today's neuroscience such terms as cate-cholamin*ergic* and peptid*ergic*.

This sort of thing could quickly get out of hand. A much more satisfactory and logical classification of neuroactive molecules is based on *messenger systems*. The *first messenger* is the substance or substances released externally onto the neuron by a presynaptic ending close to the postsynaptic membrane containing the transmitter receptor molecules. The first messenger of the system could well be acetyl choline or serotonin.

The *second messengers* are defined as molecules or ions acting as functional links between the molecular receptors in the postsynaptic membrane which respond to the neurotransmitter (first messenger) and molecular effector mechanisms (such as metabolic processes, ion pumps, ion channels or genes). A list of some identified second messengers is given in Table 1.1.

Intracellular calcium ion exists in the free form in a low and a tightly controlled concentration. Free Ca^{2+} has been referred to as *the ion of explosive*

Table 1.1 Second messenger systems of neuron and their probable role[*]

Ion or molecule	Function
Calcium in free ionic form (Ca^{2+})	Initiation of a cascade of enzyme reactions in a cell
cyclic AMP	Formed from ADP by the action of adenylate cyclase
The G-protein system	Promotion of cAMP formation
A phospholipid component of the neuron membrane (phosphatidylinositol)	Releasing Ca in the bound or sequestered form to free ionic Ca^{2+}
Cell reactions involving protein phosphorylation and methylation	The synthetis of neurotransmitter molecules

[*]Selected examples are discussed further in the text.

action. Such diverse activities as triggering of the enzyme cascade involving the coagulation of blood to the linking of excitable membrane changes to the mechanics of action of muscle fibres are but two of several. The appearance of transients of free Ca^{2+} in cells, including neurons and muscle fibres, usually presages some spectacular event.

Free Ca^{2+} in the cytoplasm, axoplasm or sarcoplasm is controlled precisely. The endoplasmic reticulum and the sarcoplasmic reticulum have ion pumps as component molecules of their membranes which are capable of sequestering (setting apart) Ca^{2+} inside the intracellular chambers (*cisternae*) of the hollow, reticular tubule system. The molecular biology of Ca^{2+} in its free and bound forms has been clearly described by Campbell (1983). The importance of matching the duration and frequency of electrical stimulation of skeletal muscle will be discussed in Chapter 8, Section 8.4. It is advisable to match the patterns of duration and frequency used during the application of electrotherapy to measurements by electromyography which have been made of the natural frequency and duration of firing of motor unit action potentials throughout normal movements.

The membranes of the sarcoplasmic reticulum contain an effective Ca^{2+} pump (Ca^{2+}/Mg^{2+} regulated ATPase) (refer to Chapter 3 for a discussion of other ion pumps which are ATPases). Release of quanta of Ca^{2+} is linked to action currents generated by action potentials and, through the second messenger action, to metabolic processes of the cell. The molecular nature of channel molecules regulating intracellular free Ca^{2+} is illustrated schematically in Fig. 1.13.

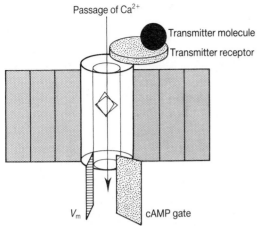

Passage of Ca²⁺

Transmitter molecule

Transmitter receptor

V_m cAMP gate

Fig. 1.13 A schematic representation of a membrane molecule which is able to control the entry of free Ca^{2+} ions into a neuron. The longitudinal shaded structures are protein components of the cell membrane. The diagonally shaded flap is a voltage controlled gate (V_m) which can be modulated by cAMP. The cylindrical channel is guarded by a neurotransmitter operated gate.

One way in which the second messenger activity is effected in the neuron is by the mediation of calcium activated neutral proteases (CANPs). The concentration of Ca^{2+} required to activate the family of CANPs divides them into defined functional groups (Zimmerman and Schlaepfer, 1984). For example, the enzymes requiring a very low concentration of free Ca^{2+} inside the cell, of the order of micromolar (μM) dimension, are referred to as μCANPs. Whereas enzymes requiring a higher, although still low concentration, of the order of millimolar (mM), are called mCANPs.

Calcium activated neutral proteases cleave proteins by limited proteolysis yielding sizeable peptide fragments. These enzymes lead also to alteration of structure and modification of the properties of a protein. Such an activity is surely a candidate for situations where protein breakdown followed by resynthesis operate in neuromuscular plastic adaptation.

The family of CANPs existing in brain and skeletal muscle serves to couple the process of enzyme activation with the cellular event associated with a transient rise in free Ca^{2+} concentration within the cell. In such a scheme, mCANP would represent the form of enzyme perturbed in a controlled fashion to be the most selective as an agent of cell protein breakdown as a consequence of the cell's own activity (autoproteolysis). Autoproteolysis must be a very important stage in the molecular

reorganization found in plastic adaptation.

The ability of Ca^{2+} to mediate in the stage of releasing transmitter molecules from the store in synaptic terminals (see Chapter 5) is believed to be important in the control of synaptic strength by learning (Kandel, 1981). Ca^{2+}-activated ATPase serves in the presynaptic membrane as an ion pump, and the localized accumulation of Ca^{2+} in the presynaptic membrane of the terminal enhances the different stages of the learning process as it is thought of in the molecular and neurobiological scale of events. This subject will be discussed in detail in Chapter 8.

Once again it is repeated that no attempt is being made at a formal presentation of biochemistry. A gradual move in your minds is being attempted instead. We are concerned more with you gaining an appreciation of molecules which move, and indeed show variable movement. One of the most misunderstood molecules concerned with the delivery of second messages is adenosine triphosphate (ATP). Introduced by Fritz Lipmann in 1941, the concept of the *high energy bond* operating in the biochemistry of linked reactions during intermediate metabolism acted like a stimulating drug on the minds of many.

Adenosine triphosphate comprises an organic base (adenine) bonded to a pentose, a five carbon ring (ribose). Together these make up the molecule adenosine (Fig 1.14).

The adenosine molecule carries three phosphate groups which split or hydrolyse, in accordance with the following reaction:

A–P–P–P goes to A–P–P and inorganic phosphate –P

similarly,

A–P–P goes to A–P and another inorganic phosphate –P

Reference to Fig. 1.14 should make this clear. What is not usually made clear about the 'high energy bonds' is that unless they are coupled to some suitable reaction which they are able to drive, their energy is little beyond the ordinary. It is their availability to difficult and driven reactions, and their favourability in the thermodynamics of reaction which makes their energy appear high.

You might have recognized already a touch of pedantry about the list of second messengers in Table 1.1 and you would be quite right to do so. It is a suspiciously neat list. The molecular neuro-

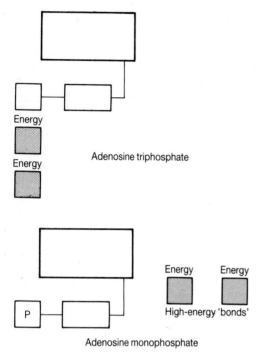

Fig. 1.14 A molecule of ATP is shown to have phosphate bonds of high energy when they are coupled to a chemical reaction which they can drive (see text). Adenosine monophosphate remains.

biological equivalent of the much loved upper and lower motoneurons of fond memory. Allow us to be not quite so precious.

Adenosine monophosphate (AMP) is not the same as cAMP (or cyclic AMP) and they should never be confused. This is shown by Fig. 1.14 in which ATP with its impressive array of P–P–P is transformed by the action of the enzyme adenylate cyclase to two moieties of inorganic phosphate (P_i) and an adenosine molecule carrying –P in ring form. Purists will recognize the difference between 3′–5′ cAMP and 5′–AMP (see Fig. 1.15).

1.7 Oh no, not another

Cyclic AMP should not be seen as a unique second messenger. Nor should it be thought of as a good 'high energy' phosphate bond carrier to have at hand. There is a class of compounds called cyclic phosphate carriers which, in terms of their molecular activity, should be called cyclic nucleotides. Cyclic AMP is but one of these. It may be that the visual acuity of prejudice is required before the glimpse of a system within a system can be

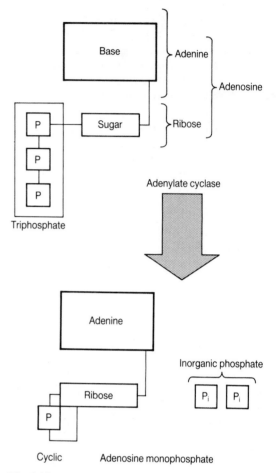

Fig. 1.15 An enzyme adenylate cyclase will split the molecule of ATP to yield two inorganic phosphate ions and cyclic AMP. This must not be confused with AMP. The phosphate group attaches to the ribose molecule at two places known as the carbon 3 and carbon 5 positions in the ring, respectively (3′-5′ AMP). This molecule belongs to the class of substances known as second messengers (see text).

resolved. The richness of interaction available in the 'stimulus–response' approach to therapy (see Chapter 6) is able to operate in the classical neurological controls. But to have that system adaptable to significant changes in environment (stimulus–stress relationships; see Chapter 1.5 above) requires a system operating within the neuromuscular system. This is the molecular system being presented.

Comb your memories for the role of acetyl choline as a neurotransmitter molecule. Released from storage in a presynaptic vesicle it diffuses across the synaptic cleft and binds (as a ligand) to the molecular receptor in the postsynaptic membrane.

Almost immediately the acetyl choline is cleaved into inactive acetyl and choline components by the enzyme *acetylcholine esterase*. Synaptic transmission is effected in that way and the synapse is cleared and ready for subsequent transmission. Making the process more general we could say:

STORE OF MOLECULES − RELEASE OF MOLECULES −
RECOGNITION OF THOSE MOLECULES −
TRANSDUCTION OF MOLECULAR CONCENTRATION
INTO AN ELECTRICAL EVENT − ENZYMATIC
DESTRUCTION OF THOSE MOLECULES

We should now be able to construct a parallel algorithm or critical path for the systems able to control neurotrophicity (cf. Chapter 7, Section 7.7). This requires the identification of a similar trinity of molecules. They can be found in the scheme that follows:

1. The synaptic transmitter molecule or possibly a hormone of the endocrine system: this may be generalized to '*a first messenger*'.

2. The membrane receptor protein to which the *first messenger* can bind as a ligand.

3. The resulting *allosteric* (allosteric translates as 'other forms') change activates a linking protein (G-protein) which moves laterally in the molecular fluidity of the neuron membrane to activate the molecule of *adenylate cyclase*.

4. The cAMP formed produces its effect as a second messenger by binding to a protein kinase which depends for its activity on the presence of cAMP liberating the catalytic component in this molecule to phosphorylate (or make active) specific membrane protein molecules effective in metabolic or physiological processes.

5. The molecule which is effective in these reactions, namely cAMP, is inactivated shortly after its action by the enzyme *phosphodiesterase* (PDE). Do you detect a similarity with what is within:

STORE OF MOLECULES − RELEASE OF MOLECULES −
RECOGNITION OF THOSE MOLECULES −
TRANSDUCTION OF MOLECULAR CONCENTRATION
INTO AN ELECTRICAL EVENT − ENZYMATIC
DESTRUCTION OF THOSE MOLECULES

There is some difference in the time course of these events which should indicate the differences between the immediacy of a response to a stimulus and the eventuality of a plastic adaptive change in response to a stress (cf. Section 1.1 above and Fig. 1.12).

A schematic illustration of a simplification of the action of the G-system is offered in Fig. 1.16. The inclusion of cGMP adds to cAMP another component of the cyclic nucleotide array which contributes to the plexus of molecular interplay in the full neurotrophic influence involved in the plastic adaptation of the central nervous system (CNS).

The roles of phosphotidyl inositol and reactions involving protein phosphorylation and methylation cannot be separated with justification.

Reference to grandmother dolls will help. The big grandmother has a smaller grandmother inside her. The small one has an even smaller grandmother tucked inside as well. All cells contain in

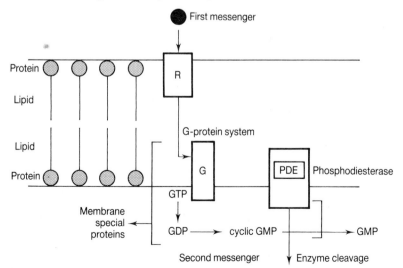

Fig. 1.16 A schematic representation of the G-protein system. This second messenger acts through the agency of special membrane proteins. It is believed to control the synthesis by the neuron of molecules during a process of plastic adaptation.

their cytoplasm a closed and interlinking tubular system. In neurons this is referred to as an *endoplasmic* reticulum. A similarly placed and structured system in muscle fibres is known as a *sarcoplasmic* reticulum. Free Ca^{2+} is removed from the cytoplasm of skeletal muscle fibres, the sarcoplasm, by its sequestration in the tubular system. Bound in this way as inactivated Ca^{2+} it is not available to trigger the molecular machines which operate in the mechanical action of skeletal muscle.

The penetration of the action currents in the muscle fibre follows the propagation of its action potential. The action currents invade the sarcoplasmic reticulum and the free Ca^{2+} so released initiates an action between actin and myosin molecules of the sarcomere.

With the endoplasmic reticulum of the neuron a similar sequestration of free Ca^{2+} takes place. But the mechanism of release is different. Phosphotidylinositol biphosphate (PIP_2) acting as a second messenger has its lipid chains cleaved by the enzyme phospholipase CC (PLC) to produce inositol triphosphate (IP_3).

This molecule releases free Ca^{2+} into the cytoplasm of the neuron from the store of bound Ca^{2+} in the endoplasmic reticulum.

1.8   Oh yes there is, and yet another one still!

The Ca^{2+} freed in this way operates as a *third messenger*, introducing into reactions a response that differs in the dimension of time from the action of free Ca^{2+} as *second messenger* discussed above. A *fourth messenger* system is trying to emerge, but for the time being we will let that system wait in the wings.

We should be getting across to you that molecular neurobiology is introducing you to a system of molecules that acts rather as a network of control

(Fig. 1.17). This network is almost as rich in its interplay as the neuronal networks of the CNS. We need some hook, though, from which to hang our developing arguments. The introduction of neuromolecular biology as a control system within a control system allows us to explore what it is that upsets the balance of neurotransmission and neuromodulation. For those of our readers who still hold a fond belief in the 'upper motoneuron and lower motoneuron' model of the CNS we suggest a few minutes in a darkened room and the application to the forehead of a cool and dampened cloth.

We owe to Otto Loewi, working in the early years of the 1900s, the idea that chemicals could possibly mediate the transmission between excitable cells. Around the same time, Langley proposed that in the autonomic nervous system a substance resembling adrenaline was released from the terminals onto effector cells in the system. Further postulates from him suggested that the *chemical link* between cells could be dependent on the *amount of nervous impulse activity* and that specific *molecular receptors* were available on the responding cells to receive and relay the activity.

In the 1930s Henry Dale demonstrated that acetylcholine was a transmitter substance in autonomic ganglia as well as at the synapse between the motoneuron terminal and muscle fibre. In its entirety the nervous system can employ a legion of different transmitter molecules. But that is not so at all of the synapses of a single neurone. Dale's principle was pithy on this point:

> . . . during development some process of differentiation determined the particular secretory product a given neuron will manufacture, store and release (at its endings). If a substance can be established as the transmitter at one synapse, it can be inferred to be the transmitter at all other synapses made by that neuron.
>
> Dale (1935)

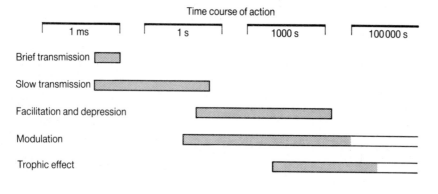

Fig. 1.17 An illustration of a comparative approach to the time course of action of neurotransmitter molecules and molecules belonging to the second messenger systems.

This was gripped by the burgeoning but somewhat uncritical minds of the time as by the jaws of a bulldog, and what was a principle written clearly became, in its loose application, a possible block to the understanding of neuromodulation.

A diversity of action exists for a transmitter released from a single neuron. A neuron with such diverse action can be referred to as a *multiaction meuron*. It was Kandel who condensed thought on this matter. He writes *inter alia*:

> The synaptic action is not detemined by the transmitter but by the properties of the receptors on the postsynaptic cell.
>
> The receptors on the postsynaptic neurons of a single presynaptic neuron can be pharmacologically distinct and can control different ionic chanels.
>
> A single postsynaptic cell may have more than one kind of receptor for a given transmitter, each receptor controlling a different ionic conductance mechanism.
>
> Kandel (1976)

This loosening of the stranglehold of the unqualified principle of Dale allows us to point out the great amplification of synaptic effect that can be obtained, as well as an additional and variable control, by a modulation of that effect.

1.9 Upper modulation and lower modulation? You must be joking

If you take the wealth of understanding that has been obtained about the classical approach to stimulus–response neurophysiology (see Chapter 6) you should now be prepared to accept that classical neurophysiology has a form of gearbox. The lever which can shift the gear from third, in which the normal nervous system drives movements, can also shift to fourth and overdrive gear ratios. It is possible also to drop the drive to the second and first gears.

The hand on the gear lever belongs to those marvellous hands illustrated in Fig. 1.1, but unfortunately there is evidence that disordered motor controls can operate also to generate modulation of synaptic activity. There is a possibility that a misunderstanding of neuromodulation lingers still in the orthodox minds of therapists.

Allow us to explain what neuromodulation *is not*. There is no equivalent scheme involving EXCITATION – INHIBITION – MODULATION. There is no equivalent, for example, of central

excitatory state (CES) and central inhibitory state (CIS). No equivalent central modulatory state exists. The interplay in a control system between CES and CIS requires a fast acting and rapidly conducting system of neurons and muscles. But the development of appropriate modulation is, by comparison, much slower than the stimulus–response type of motor system that has been so far described. This is illustrated in Fig. 1.17.

Note firstly the very great scale of time encompassed by the diagram. The brief transmission of a stimulus–response neurophysiology can be measured in the millisecond (ms) range of time. A slower transmission which usually requires some facilitation extends the time course of action to the second (s) scale of time. Neuromodulation requires a longer time to take effect and endures for much longer than is thought of in the time scales appropriate to a stimulus–response neurophysiology.

Neuromodulation does not operate over the hard wired type of circuitry suitable for CES/CIS type of neural control. The heart of neuromodulation resides in the second, third and fourth messenger systems and the way in which they modulate the macromolecular structures and location which modify the characteristics of both neuron and skeletal muscle.

1.10 If the first clear facts about the Unseen World seem small and trivial, should that deter us from the quest?

F. W. H. Myers, Human Personality

The molecular forms, localizations and activities within neurons and muscles will form the subject matter of the remainder of this book. It shall be shown, for example, that precursors of the neurotransmitter molecules of acetylcholine, which are held in vesicles of the neuromuscular junction, are formed by the motoneuron nucleus. The molecular receptor molecules which are found in the membrane of the postsynaptic neuron or muscle fibre are similarly formed. Molecules able to act as ion pumps in the neuron membrane establish the concentration of the ions Na^+ and K^+. In the endplate of skeletal muscle, voltage-dependent Ca^{2+} channels respond (see Fig. 1.13) to the action currents generated by the excitation of the synaptic endings and allow free Ca^{2+} ions to initiate the process of acetylcholine release.

A molecular approach will be made also to the

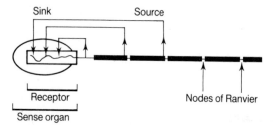

Fig. 1.18 A diagram indicating the difference between a receptor ending of an afferent axon and the sense organ in which it is found. Illustrated also is the direction of current flow from sources in the regenerative regions of the axon, to the sink generated by the transducer region of the receptor ending.

activities of the nerve-to-nerve synapse. There will be discussion of excitation, inhibition and presynaptic inhibition and placing of the modulatory actions discussed in the sections above into the scheme explaining the ways in which a synapse can be changed as a result of plastic adaptation (see Fig. 1.18).

Figure 1.20 illustrates diagrammatically the mode of response of a mechanoceptor to the application of a stretch stimulus. The mechanical stimulus has a ramp form: giving a dynamic component (as the stimulus *is being applied*) followed by a static component (as the stimulus *is maintained steadily*). A generator potential develops which is localized to the patches of sensory molecules in the membrane of the sense organ (see Fig. 1.19).

The ghost of a stimulus–response neurophysiology should now be laid forever (only to find it resur-

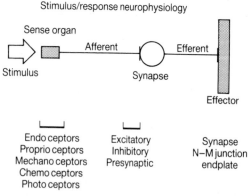

Fig. 1.19 A diagram of a simple reflex arc to show the various parts of it that can be explained in terms of the molecules discussed in molecular neurobiology. The classical names are retained. Stimulus–response physiology stops where this diagram starts. Sherrington was responsible for the *ceptor* classification of sensory receptor endings.

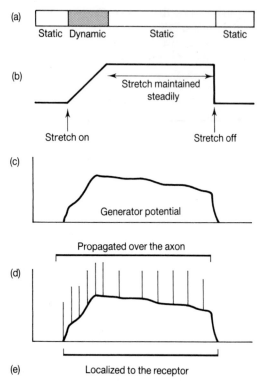

Fig. 1.20 A summary of the electrical activity of a sensory receptor. A localized, non-propagated and graded potential is generated by the stimulated sensory receptor ending. Action potentials initiated in the afferent axon in response to this are all-or-nothing and propagated towards the CNS. This sensory mechanoceptor signals the *significance* of the stimulus to the ongoing motor activity at the time.

rected in Chapter 6 as a careful justification of our thoughts on neuromuscular plasticity). Bell, book and candle will then be exhibited just in case any of our readers are clinging still to the comfort of familiarity.

The days of the Organ of Ruffini, the Disc of Merkel and the Corpuscle of Pacini are past, but remembered with respect still in the archives of history. Very much alive today and kicking vigorously is the classification of *ceptors* made by Sherrington (Fig. 1.19). The sensory receptors are transducers in that they change the form of energy obtained in the stimulus and make it recognizable, for example, as an electric current flow, to the afferent neuron of a reflex arc. Thus endoceptors change the energy of a particular stimulus internal to the body fluid compartments into a local depolarization of the excitable patches of membrane in the sensory receptor. The sense organ with a speciali-

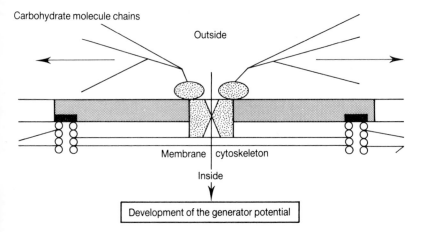

Carbohydrate molecule chains

Outside

Membrane | cytoskeleton

Inside

Development of the generator potential

Fig. 1.21 A schematic illustration of the molecular structure of one of the mechanoceptor regions in the membrane of a sensory neuron. The forces generated by stretching are transmitted to the transducer molecule by molecular strands in both the internal and external components of the membrane. The ion flow initiated in this way develops the generator potential (see Fig. 1.20 and the text).

zed capsule matches the energy of the stimulus to the sensitivity of the energy absorbing molecules of the receptor. We should specify that we are writing here of sensory receptors and not of transmitter receptor molecules of the postsynaptic membrane of the neuron and neuromuscular junctions.

The effector structures of the reflex arc will be, in the argument of this book, the skeletal muscle fibres and they will be looked upon, as it progresses, as an assembly of molecules that are able to carry out the metabolism to energize the molecules of muscle mechanical action: the several forms of molecule including and operating with actin and myosin.

The nerve-to-nerve synapse of the reflex arc contains a wealth of protein molecules essential for its action. Precursors of the molecules of transmission, as we have written, may be synthesized in the neuron soma and travel by axonal transport down the length of the efferent axon.

The electrical components of a simplified mechanoceptor are shown in Fig. 1.20. The *sensory receptor ending* is a modified length of the afferent axon contained within the capsule of the *sensory receptor organ*. Please note the distinction of receptor ending from receptor organ in that definition. The development of a localized and non-propagated generator potential acts as a *sink* for current to flow into from nearby *sources* of current at the regeneration zones (e.g. nodes of Ranvier) at points along the afferent axon.

The transduction of stimulus energy is also shown in Fig. 1.20. A stimulus in the form of stretch applied to a mechanoceptor is shown by its moving or dynamic component (Figs 1.20a and b). The molecules transducing the energy develop a gener-

ator potential which acts as a current *sink* (see Fig. 1.20). The receptor membrane of the sensor measures the *significance of the stimulus* to motor activity underway. It is this measure of *significance* which is coded into an action potential train which is propagated by the afferent axon towards the CNS. At the sensory receptor ending, the separate electrical events of generator and action potentials add or summate (Fig. 1.20d). The slow and graded generator potential is localized to the receptor (Fig. 1.20e) whereas the action potentials are propagated over the afferent axon (Fig. 1.20d).

Adopting a schematic illustration of the complex protein molecules which form a sensory receptor site in the axonal membrane (see Fig. 1.21) the transducer molecule detects the mechanical forces that are coupled to it (stippled) by two structures: (1) strands in the form of carbohydrate molecules running over the outside of the membrane, and (2) the filaments of the internal skeleton of the neuron (cytoskeleton) running along the inside surface of the membrane. The resulting movement of ions across the membrane generates an area at the point of mechanical action into which ionic current can *sink*. It is the flow from the *source* of ionic current that encodes the action potential train propagated towards the CNS.

References

Dale, H. H. (1935). *Pharmacology and nerve endings*. Pro. Roy. Soc. Med. **28**; 319–332

Dyson, R. D. (1974). *Cell Biology. A molecular approach*. Allyn and Bacon, Boston, U.S.A.

Kandel, E. R. (1976). *Cellular basis of behaviour*. W. H. Freeman, San Francisco.

Sherrington, C. S. (1904). *The correlation of reflexes and the principle of the common final path*. Brit. Ass. **74**; 728–744.

Chapter 2

An introduction to cellular neurobiology

2.1 The difference between molecular and cellular neurobiology

The relationship between the complex structure of different macromolecules has been introduced in Chapter 1. A recapitulation of the dynamics of their structure will be offered here and in Chapters 3, 5, 7 and 8. Neuromuscular rehabilitation requires you to distinguish the subtleties between complexity and improbability, between stability and mutability, between life and being alive, between dying and dead.

Starting to assemble in discussion, as we have done, a series of molecules of ascending complexity until we touched upon the characteristics of improbability, we must now begin to perform the operation in reverse. Starting with the neuron, we will indulge in a little *reductionism*, where the telling argument is that 'the sum of the parts is greater than the whole' whereas, we will argue elsewhere, with equal cogency, that *holism* rules. Holism states that 'the whole is greater than the sum of its parts'. If you are sufficiently open minded to accept that the neuromuscular system is plastic, you will have no difficulty reconciling the two dissimilar philosophies. In so doing you will realize that the movement forwards of rehabilitation has been held back by a professional reaction, and that it will be released and progress further just as soon as we are comfortable in our minds with REDUCTIONISMWHOLEISM as we are about the realism of FORMFUNCTION (cf. Introduction and Chapter 7).

There is a species of label, intended to be fastened to the inside of a motor car window, which says ESCHEW OBFUSCATION: unfortunately, this message is often concealed by grime. It is time possibly to do a bit of eschewing of obfuscation in this book. We have seen how the plasma membrane of a neuron can be resolved to molecules representing patches of life contained in an arguably none-alive matrix of simpler molecules. An improbability, which approaches that of J. Z. Young's definition of life (referred to above), is given by the allosteric changes that the molecules can make. Even the non-alive matrix of molecules shows an improbability of a stable structure, in the molecular context, by its fluidity and readiness to allow molecules to be inserted into itself and move around within itself.

When a cellular neurobiology is compared with a complementary molecular neurobiology the two disciplines are seen as being separated by only a whisker of reasoning. It is interesting to note the way in which the contemporary neuroscience is using more and more the location of the molecules of neurochemical importance as a source of distinction between neurons and between neuronal systems (cf. Shepherd 1979, 1988).

The gradual but irresistible change of terminology again highlights the congruities within cellular neurobiology and molecular neurobiology. We intend to develop this approach to our subject fully in the following section.

2.2 Eponimics have had their day

We intend no disrespect to the scholars who equipped our science with academic respectability, but we must present the coherence of disciplines that have given rise to the scientific, clinical rehabilitation we are presenting. The cells of Betz and Purkinje live still as do the nucleus of Deiter and the column of Clarke. Medical students reel to this day at the *Substantia gelatanosa Rolandi*, and the *iter a tertio ad quartem ventriculum* generates a fear that is disproportionate to its anatomical size.

Two newer classifications of neuronal systems deserve mention. The first concerns itself with the *ergic* quality of the system concerned. This quality concerns itself with the chemical nature of the neurotransmitter conveying information through the division of the nervous system in which it is involved. Two of the neurotransmitter classifications are presented in detail in Chapter 1. They are the *cholinergic* and *adrenergic* divisions of the autonomic nervous system. The presence of the two transmitters is accompanied by genetically determined enzymes which inactivate them. They are, respectively, acetylcholine esterase and monoamine oxidase, the transmitters acetylcholine and noradrenaline. Other *ergic* systems involving distinct populations of neurons are presented as Table 2.1

A remarkable development in neurobiology over recent years has been the recognition of the widespread distribution of neuroactive peptides. Almost as remarkable has been the insight of the research workers involved and the flexibility of their minds to see an unusual system developing. Over 50 neuroactive peptides exist in the brain with putative neuroactive peptides reaching a number of 100

or more. There is in fact no definitive list available. A recent review by Cooper *et al.* (1987) evoked a comment from the authors: 'we write with pencil in one hand and an eraser in the other'!

The development of neuropeptide physiology gives a clear indication that the borderline between the nervous and endocrine systems is becoming indistinct. The identity of what is known as the gut–brain system can be seen from Table 2.1. The embryological origins of these endocrine/neuro-active molecules can be observed also from their description as an APUD system: 'the system of **a**mine **p**recursor, **u**ptake and **d**ecarboxylation'.

The gut–brain hormones (see again Table 2.1) are believed to play a part in the hunger–satiety behavioural axis. In 1975, biochemical studies revealed that there are molecular receptors in the brain and spinal cord that bind specifically to morphine, a substance that is both pain-killing and addictive. The question of whether or not the central nervous system (CNS) evolved receptors just to bind the molecule of morphine, or developed possibly the receptors to bind endogenous morphine-like molecules (endorphins) was soon answered. Two small molecules, in the pentapeptide range of size, were isolated from brain extracts. They were named enkephalins. Eventually, the chemical isolation of different opioid peptides

Table 2.1 Classification of neural systems into the type of neurotransmitter.

Transmitter	Type of system	Activity
Acetylcholine	Cholinergic	Neuromuscular transmission, parasympathetic transmission
Adrenalin	Adrenergic	Hormone
Nor-adrenalin	Nor-adrenergic	Sympathetic non–synaptic transmission, transmission in the somatic nervous system
Dopamine	Dopaminergic	Psychogenic activity
Serotonin	Serotoninergic	Modulation of mood
Amino acids	Aminergic	
Gamma aminobutyrate		Inhibition
Glutamate glycine		Excitatory transmission, inhibitory adjuvant
Neuroactive peptides	Peptidergic	
Carnosine		
TRH		
Met enkephalin		
Leu enkephalin		
Oxytocin		
Vasopressin		
LHRH	Refer to the text	
Substance P		
Neurotensin		
Somatosin		
VIP		
Beta endorphin		
ACTH		

revealed a powerful apparatus of neuropeptides which was important from both purely scientific and clinical points of view.

Taking a different approach to the brain, it was estimated in a quantitative approach to neuronal population (see Chapter 5) that the approximate number of neurons in the human brain is 10 000 000 000 (10 billion). Each neuron within this population is estimated as making 10 000 contacts with other neurons: giving 100 trillion synaptic connections in all. Neurons are various in their form and great confusion can arise from an unqualified mix of classical and descriptive names. The cell body or soma of the neuron surrounds the nucleus and is defined as doing so. The nucleus is the centre of metabolic control of the neuron and its processes. The main organelles of the neuron are found in the soma also. This structural relationship allows them to interact with each other and with the nucleus. The growth during neurogenesis and maturation of neuronal specialization carries some of the soma organelles out to peripheral locations. Mitochondria and vesicles filled with transmitter molecules are two such organelles found in synaptic terminals.

Next to be considered are the neuronal processes or branches. The pattern of branching in neurons attracts pictorial and artistic names. Think of mossy fibres in the cerebellar cortex and the climbing fibres in the same structure. Shepherd (1979, 1988) introduces a form of classification for neurons that is commendably clean, even if it does take some of the magic away from neuroanatomy.

Some neurons are called principal neurons, or possibly projection or relay neurons. Typically, these neurons have a single, long process arising in an axon hillock seen as a differentiated part of the soma. They tend to make connection with distant parts of the CNS or, in the case of motoneurons, with peripheral skeletal muscle fibres. In Shepherd's classification the processes known as dendrites are all those branches that do not fulfil the criteria needed to be called an axon. Within the neuronal sphere of interaction there are neurons with shorter axons. These are classified as interneurons or intrinsic neurons. This last name is more suitable when it is used to describe the limits of a *set* of neurons which have a distinct function (see Chapter 4). Any neuron with a soma outside a recognizable set but whose terminals end within a set are considered to be afferent to that set.

Some neurons are so small that an axon cannot

be distinguished from the other processes. These are known either as amacrine or anaxonal neurons or more loosely as granule cells. A great deal of time has been employed since Sherrington (1906) published his *Integrative Action of the Nervous System* and put into scientific usage the terms and definitions that so clarified the original stages of understanding the nervous system. We hope that the use of that time to add a molecular dimension to the subject is not an arrogance and that it offers an even more unifying approach to an already integrated nervous action.

2.3   A glimpse . . .

Homo sapiens has the neural equipment to classify itself amongst the higher animals, and it does so. We belong, to be exact, to the class known as *eukaryotes* in which a specialization of organelles, for example, mitochondria, centrioles, microfilaments and microtubules, amongst others, exists in the cytoplasm of their cells. An organelle, separated from the cytoplasm by a membrane, the nuclear envelope, is the nucleus which bears the chromosomes consisting of DNA and associated proteins. It is best to think of the nature of the nuclear envelope in the way in which we introduced the nature of the membranes bounding other fluid compartments of the body (Chapter 1).

The two 'polythene bag' model, in which the largest and innermost holds the intracellular phase is no longer sufficient on its own. Another 'polythene bag' holding the interstitial fluid phase and separating from it the circulating phase, the plasma, adds to the model the properties of selective permeability and semipermeability.

A porous nuclear membrane (the 'polythene bag' which contains DNA and associated protein) allows the transcription of units of information contained in DNA into ribose nucleic acid (RNA). The DNA, of course, is the master copy from which duplicates are prepared during cell division (mitosis), growth and development, and in the processes of repair. Mitotic activity is essential to the functioning of neurons and many other cells. This function is present in the CNS during development but is lost, or not naturally available, in most mature neurons. Notable exceptions in neurobiology are found in the olfactory receptor neuron in vertebrates and some neurons of the brain centres controlling bird song.

All that we have ever been, what we are now and

what we could possibly be in the future is held in store by the genome (see Fig. 2.1). This is the genetic complement, formed by the fusion of haploid gametes from both parents, ranged along the chromosomes which are central to the control of life processes in every cell of the body. We are said to have a genome composed of 100 000 genes (see Chapter 5). If we can picture the *curriculum vitae* of the human at a cellular level we would refer to it as the genotype of that particular individual. Imagine the genes representing the genotype as folders in a filing cabinet. Some of them are covered in dust: they are the genes which have not attracted the attention of the environment and remain unexpressed. Other genes, or other folders in the filing cabinet, are well thumbed: they are genes that respond to an effective change in environment.

This, the sum of characteristics manifested by an organism, is referred to as the phenotype. Contrast this with the full set of genes possessed by it; in other words contrast it with the genotype. In rehabilitation of the neuromuscular system our concern is with the genes expressed in response to a change in environment. Environmentally determined, or let's face up to it, a therapeutically determined gene expression, will order differently the molecular distribution and activity at the adapting sites of nerve and muscle. Yours are, most certainly, the most marvellous of hands!

Our definition of plasticity, particularly that of the neuromuscular system, needs a little refinement. The adaptation of nerve and muscle does not have a 'flip-flop' character. It is not a matter of *now you see it, now you don't.* It is a process of life which is in continuous operation. Figure 2.2 attempts an illustration of this. The environmental change demanding adaptation operates on the state of the system: in this case the neuromuscular system. Not the state of just one part of it: the state of all of it. This starts the *wheel of state* spinning until a further justification of statement FORMFUNCTION appears as the two separate parts of the word fuse together and cannot be recognized separately.

Cellular neurobiology takes into full account that the whole is greater than the sum of its parts by not recognizing one cell, or if it comes to that, one molecule. This is done just as naturally as a gar-

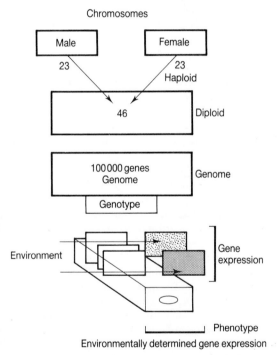

Fig. 2.1 The complement of genes carried by the chromosomes in the nucleus of each of our cells is estimated as being 100 000. This number is known as the genome. The chromosomes are formed by the result of fusion of haploid germ cells. Our *curriculum vitae*, in this respect, gives our genotype and represents our potentiality. What we are, as opposed to what we could be, is given by the number of folders taken carefully from our filing cabinet of genes. This is our phenotype. A significant change in environment expresses some genes apart from others, this activity is referred to as a form of environmentally determined gene expression. Neuromuscular plasticity depends on this.

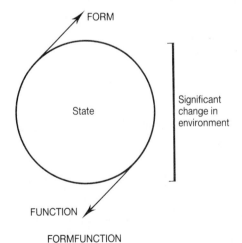

Fig. 2.2 A significant change in environment alters the state of a cell (or cells or tissues or organs). The initially identifiable and separate FORM and FUNCTION blur as the 'wheel of state' begins to revolve. An inseparable FORMFUNCTION remains.

dener would not recognize that there was just one greenfly on a rose bush. Reference to Fig. 2.3 will make this clear. Two neurons in contact (the poached egg appearance is intentional with much more attention paid to axonal and dendritic processes in Chapters 3 and 8) are much more information-rich than the two neurons thought of separately.

Acronyms can defeat their own purpose but some, however, are useful. There is an acronym which describes well the dysentery experienced by incautious tourists in Africa. It is WAWA: which means that wily Africa wins again. Two neurons communicate each with the other by synthesis of membrane component molecules called NCAM.

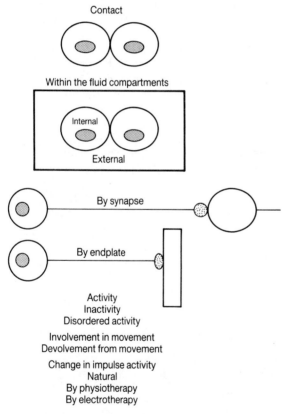

Fig. 2.3 Contact between contiguous cells gives the opportunity of mutual control. This control is enhanced if it is carried out in humoral or hormonal environment in the body fluids. The poached egg shapes are intentional, but when the processes of axon are admitted, synaptic and endplate points of connection add other features of control. Activity will be shown to be important in plastic adaptation, and activity contains the elements listed at the bottom of the figure.

This represents 'nerve cell adhesion molecules'. An approximation of two neurites causes the expression of genes, in one or both, which direct the synthesis and placement in the membranes of this agent. In what sounds very much like a developing infatuation, each tastes the other to explore the feasibility of a functional connection.

Seeming not to be able to loosen an idea we should now at least doff our caps to the large proteoglycan molecule as a component of the membrane of the developing neuron. It is called NILE (nerve growth factor induced large external glycoprotein) and is again an adhesion molecule. However, the ambiguous acronym could be redolent of WAWA and it is better left to the sympathetic treatment of Chapter 8.

An extension of this thinking to include our two developing neurons interacting within and around the fluid compartments admits the possible (see Chapters 3 and 8) signalling between the two by paracrene, endocrine and humoral agents. More realistic than the poached egg approach are the two diagrams at the bottom of the series of Fig. 2.3.

Thinking of synaptic connection, both in the sense of nerve-to-nerve synapses and nerve-to-muscle synapses (both will be treated in Chapter 4) shows the wealth of interaction that is possible when the concepts within cellular neurobiology are applied in full.

A considerable proportion of this book will be devoted to activity-induced plastic adaptation of the neuromuscular system (Chapter 7). We must therefore take on board in our arguments, as well as the factors of neuronal congruity we have just outlined, the variants of activity listed as the remaining part of Fig. 2.3 and the frightening admission of the possibility that disordered activity, which we are attempting to suppress, is itself capable of engendering adaptation of the neuromuscular system to suit its own purposes. That possibility will go away if we switch on the 'blessed light of reason' and feed the meter with the coin of facts we have just outlined. The light then will not go out too soon.

The ghoulies and ghosties and the things that go bump in the night will fade also before that light, and so will the situation illustrated by Fig. 2.4. It has been said elsewhere 'if it is alive it is plastic; if it is not plastic, it is dead'. Similarly, and straight from the shoulder, Chapter 5 admonishes us to 'use it or lose it'. We are convinced by now that you will determine, with certainty, that all of the adap-

Activity
Inactivity
Disordered activity
Involvement in movement
Devolvement from movement
Change in impulse activity
Natural
By physiotherapy
By electrotherapy

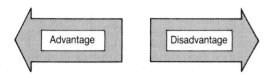

Fig. 2.4 The set-up of Fig. 2.3 is repeated with the caution that plastic adaptation is unavoidable in life. This must be recognized and care taken to direct it to the advantage of the patient.

tations your therapies bring about will progress to the advantage of your patients. Plastic adaptation of the neuromuscular system, in one direction or the other, just has to take place, there is no alternative.

We have seen, as a glimpse, that the informational content of DNA lies with its sequence of bases. Information in that form may be transferred to messenger RNA (mRNA). The translation of units of length of DNA into a series of mRNA molecules forms a series of 'templates' from which the molecules to be employed during neuromolecular rehabilitation can be recognized and assembled during synthesis. We will restrict our discussion of this particular facet of genetics to events important to neurons.

The biochemists James Watson and Francis Crick demonstrated in 1953 that a polymer called deoxyribose nucleic acid or alternatively DNA, the now famous double helix, has paired strands which lie in relationship with each other in an 'antiparallel' fashion. That interrelationship can be described simply as one strand having a sequence of: carbon number 5 to phosphate to carbon number 3 (in the convention of biochemistry: $-5'$ carbon-phosphate $-3'$ carbon). Whereas the other strand has a 'backbone' with the subtle difference of $3'$ carbon–phosphate–$5'$ carbon. The organic bases of the nucleotides are stacked in pairs at the centre of the length of the helices, with the plane of the bases perpendicular to the helix pair. The two strands are tied together by hydrogen bonds (see Chapter 1, Section 1.1), two

bonds between each adenine–thymine pair (A =T) and three between each guanine–cytosine pair (G≡C). The sequence of events involved in the transcription of DNA into RNA is illustrated simply by Fig. 2.5.

The history of RNA has been less dramatic than that for DNA. The molecules of RNA are not in fact considered as a component of the neuron nucleus: rather as molecules shuttling between nucleus and cytosol by way of the nuclear pores. Three classes of RNA exist in the neuron: mRNA, ribosomal RNA (rRNA) and transfer RNA (tRNA). You may see this latter class called soluble RNA or, as you must have guessed, sRNA.

2.4 A long, hard stare . . .

Although the path of the research followed by Crick and Watson was a biochemistry of great insight, an earlier study in the 1940s by Beadle and Tatum held the developing mind of one of us. Stripped to the bone of the argument, a protein molecule D could be formed from the pool of available amino acids A through intermediate stages B and C, with all of the reactions being influenced respectively by the enzymes, E^1 E^2 and E^3. Beadle and Tatum noticed that a genetic mutation could effect one from each of the three enzymes. This observation gave rise to the 'one gene = one enzyme' hypothesis. Actually, the hypothesis is true only in a limited sense. As the knowledge of enzyme structure developed it was realized that many enzymes are composed from more than a single polypeptide chain, and that a single mutation may affect one type of chain without affecting the others. But a similar elegance in thinking accepts that genes do not only make enzymes: they make other protein molecules also. With the remarkable realization that although genes do not always make proteins, most of them do so and that amongst those proteins are the simple and conjugated proteins responsible for the molecular modification associated with plastic adaptation.

The genome of the human cell has available within it the codes required for transcription of proteins from the past, for the present and just waiting for you: the therapists born again to understand the biochemistry of rehabilitation. No, that is a lie. The genome has mechanisms for producing proteins of novel action, and devices for amplifying the genes required to do just that. But first we must look more closely at the theory.

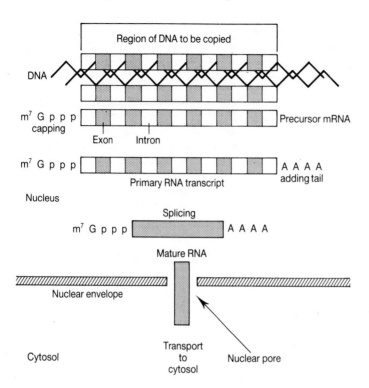

Fig. 2.5 Copies of parts of the information carried on DNA is made into mRNA. At early stages in mRNA the molecule is capped and tailed to prevent it interacting with cell dynamics too soon. Another and similar safeguard is the punctuation of the code carrying strips, the exons, by lengths of intron which are neutral in the sense of carrying no information. With all exons spliced together and the introns removed the activated, tailless and capless mRNA escapes the nucleus, enters the cytosol and becomes available for action in biosynthesis.

We suppose the word 'gene' was perfectly adequate for the enunciation of early genetic theory. Now we must look critically at our vocabulary and find some word more suitable. Some of us lost sleep when the 'one gene = one enzyme' hypothesis floundered. But morning light soon came with the replacement of 'gene' by *cistron*. A cistron is a gene defined functionally, i.e. a length of DNA producing the mRNA molecules that in turn direct the production of specific polypeptide chains that function in defined processes within the neuron.

Figure 2.5 illustrates a series of points we require for further discussion. The figure is highly diagrammatic and makes no pretence at the realities of scale. The length of DNA to be copied into RNA molecules, which are then joined together or polymerized, is shown at the top of the diagram. The cistron is copied below and becomes a precursor RNA of the sort used in sending messages or information to regions of protein synthesis in the cytosol. It is therefore messenger RNA or mRNA.

In the first stage of transcription, and whilst the mRNA is still inside the nucleus, the eventual coding regions of the mRNA (the exons) are spaced by non-coding regions (the introns). Immediately the transcription is completed in the nucleus, one end of the maturing mRNA is 'capped' with a methylated guanosine molecule (more exactly, in this context, called a molecule that is part of another molecule). In other words a residue is added to the (number 5) 5′ end of the RNA by means of a triphosphate bridge (m^7 G p p p 5′ is the notation for that process). It signals to the structures used eventually for synthesis (the ribosome) at which end of the mRNA molecule the polypeptide synthesis is to be initiated. This structure, the ribosome, will be discussed in more detail below. When transcription of mRNA in the nucleus has ended a 'tail' is added to the molecule to complement the 'cap'. The tail, a chain of adenylate molecules (A) is added to the 3′ end of the mRNA. This poly-A tail may contain as many as 200 adenylate residues. The functioning of the poly-A tail is unclear but it is hypothesized that the mRNA lacking a tail is important for the development of nerve cells. It is absent in the foetus; the population of tail carrying molecules appears shortly after birth, but it does not reach its maximum until young adulthood is reached. The punctuation marks of introns are removed from the text of exons by the procedure of splicing the exons of the polymer of mRNA, and it becomes mature.

The mature mRNA, still bearing splendidly its cap and tail, is next transported to the cytosol, passing though the nuclear pore in the nuclear envelope. It is then able to act with the other types of RNA and begin the formation of polypeptide molecules.

2.5 Nucleolus is *not* the diminutive of nucleus

The top of Fig. 2.6 starts where Fig. 2.5 ended. This figure includes two bodies (the nucleoli) which are small by comparison with the nucleus. This does not mean that the name 'nucleolus' should be taken as meaning 'a small nucleus'. The nucleoli are included in this diagram to emphasize their close involvement with the other two related structures: the polysome and ribosomes ranged along a length of endoplasmic reticulum and giving it a roughened appearance under the microscope.

Following synthesis from a DNA template in the nucleolus, the molecules of the rRNA are first formed as a small and a large subunit. These become immediately joined together and, in combination with accessory protein components, the ribosomes leave the nucleus via the nuclear pore and reach the cytosoplasm (cytosol). The proteins involved with the nucleus and the nucleolus are formed in the cytoplasm, so there is a shuttling traffic of molecules passing through the nuclear pore. Arriving in the cytoplasm, the ribosomes are sorted into two populations: one of which remains free within the cytoplasm, either singly or as clusters of single ribosomes aggregated as granular polyribosomes. The other population is attached to the endoplasmic reticulum and is bound there in orderly sequence. The endoplasmic reticulum extends throughout the cytoplasm of cells as a basketwork or network of interlinking tubules. Taking sometimes the form of small canals, hollow sheets, membrane enclosed spaces (cysternae) or small spaces known as vacuoles, the endoplasmic reticulum may be compared with the sarcoplasmic reticulum found specifically in striated muscle fibres.

The nucleolus serves additionally to amplify the successive copying onto mRNA molecules of one copy made from the master held in the chromosome. The mRNA cistrons are linearly repeated along a chromosome in a region known as the *nuclear organizer*. The nuclear organizer is a cistron which represents 450 repeated genes and it is powerful in programming for the repertoire of the neurons during rehabilitation. Gene amplification

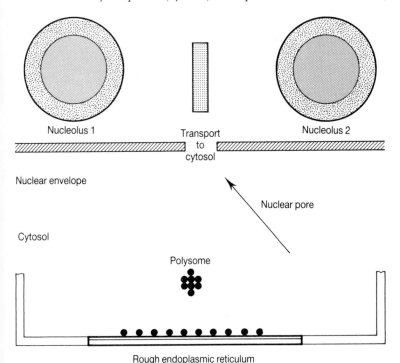

Nucleolus 1

Transport to cytosol

Nucleolus 2

Nuclear envelope

Cytosol

Nuclear pore

Polysome

Rough endoplasmic reticulum

Fig. 2.6 Starting where we left off in Fig. 2.5, the mRNA can be amplified by the nucleoli and react on the surface of ribosomes. These surfaces are formed from many ribosomes occurring as a granule in the cytosol or as ribosomes ranged along a strip of the surface of the endoplasmic reticulum.

can be seen therefore as a process instrumental in
the rapid reproduction of protein molecules. These
are needed to meet the extensive neuronal and muscular modification required during repair or
rehabilitation.

The fleet of RNA molecules is almost fully
described. Review of the story so far may be made
by reference to Fig. 2.7. Referring, for the sake of
simplicity, to one strand of the double strand of
DNA. The genetic code, which is able to determine
the sequence in which amino acids are polymerized
to form a protein, is composed from the nucleotide
bases which give DNA its uniqueness. Three adjacent nucleotides or more specifically their bases
form one unit in the code. This is called the codon.
The sequence of guanine-cytosine-adenine (or
G-C-A) is the codon for the amino acid alanine.

The necessary intermediary of action between
rRNA and mRNA is transfer RNA (tRNA). This
is a relatively small molecule of about 80 nucleotides and has a size of 25 000 amu or daltons. Before
an amino acid can be incorporated into a lengthening chain of a polypeptide molecule it must be first
'activated' by esterification and linking to tRNA.
That event is catalysed by the enzyme aminoacyl-
tRNA synthetase.

The sequence of nucleotides G–T–A–C . . . in
the single strand of DNA (Fig. 2.7, upper part)
attracts to itself a complementary strand
C–A–T–G. . . . The formation of the second polymer leads to its linking by weak bonds to the first.

The development of mRNA starts when the
nucleotides are attracted to their complement in an
opened single strand and nucleotides in succession
are polymerized or joined together by the enzyme
RNA polymerase. So we have two of the necessary
three RNA types: rRNA and mRNA. The final one
needed is tRNA. A molecule of tRNA is able to
activate a specific amino acid. A simple flow chart
of the process is:

$$\text{Amino acid (aa)} + \text{ATP} + \text{Activating enzyme}$$
$$\text{(E)} = \text{(aa–AMP–E)} + \text{PP}_i \qquad (1)$$

followed by

$$\text{(aa–AMP–E)} + \text{tRNA} = \text{aa–tRNA} +$$
$$\text{E} + \text{AMP} \qquad (2)$$

where aa–AMP–E is the activated amino acid, and
the procedure of activation employs the bond
energy of ATP in the presence of the amino acid
and the enzyme aminoacyl–tRNA synthetase to
drive the reaction to the right with the formation

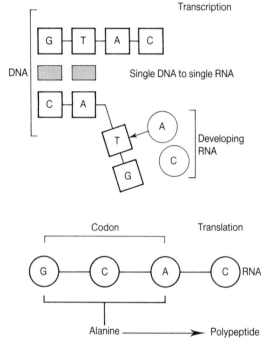

Fig. 2.7 A messenger RNA is transcribed from the genetic
code along a strand of DNA. When the mRNA is developed, it
is translated to a polypeptide (see text and Fig. 2.8).

of the activated amino acid aa–tRNA available for
assembly in the polypeptide chain. It follows that
there must be at least one activating enzyme for
each different amino acid used during the synthesis.

The amino-acid–tRNA complex (the activated
amino acid) is positioned at an mRNA molecule by
matching a three-nucleotide anticodon of the tRNA
with the corresponding codon of the messenger. In
this way, the new amino acid is brought into the
correct position with respect to the last amino acid
to be joined to the lengthening chain. The simplest
of illustrations of this event is presented as Fig. 2.7.
It shows, again diagrammatically, the process of
development on mRNA as a copy is taken of the
information carried as a master on a single strand
of DNA.

The 'activated' amino acid is carried by tRNA
(see Equation 2 above). The codon of a triplet of
nucleotides G–C–A signifies that the amino acid
carried is alanine and the tRNA molecule 'recognizes' the site on the mRNA that will accept it.

Reference to Fig. 2.8 will explain one of the
simpler processes involved in the lengthening of a
polypeptide chain during synthesis. We have no

(a)

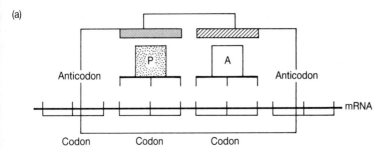

(b)

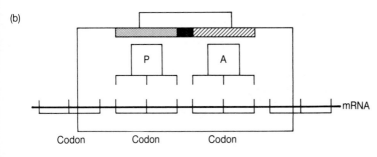

(c) Lengthening of molecular chain

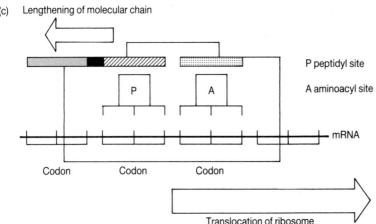

Fig. 2.8 A polypeptide chain is formed from activated amino acids recognized and carried by tRNA to mRNA. By codon/anticodon matching an exact copy from the original length of DNA is made (see text for further detail).

intention of putting in front of you more than the minimum of biochemistry needed to explain the molecular manipulation you will be invited to handle professionally as a molecular process in rehabilitation. You may forgive a simplistic analogy. A knitting pattern is borrowed and photocopied furtively before being returned. A knitting machine assembles the sock of polypeptide from the knitting pattern copy you have provided.

The first step in the production of a polypeptide chain, casting on as it were, is when two different activated amino acids carried by two different molecules of tRNA align with a ribosome in a codon--

anticodon match. This occurs at the top of Fig. 2.8. One amino acid has as its symbol a dotted rectangle, the other is diagonally hatched. The first amino acid is attached to a specific site on the ribosome referred to as the peptidyl site (P) whilst the other occupies an aminoacyl site (A). At this stage the amino acids are still unbonded.

A peptide bond is then established between the two amino acids (the filled rectangle). Translocation of the dipeptide, as it is now called, frees the tRNA from the P site and the one at the A site takes its place. This translocation frees the A site allowing another aa–tRNA (active aminoacyl–

tRNA) to take up its place and be entered next in the lengthening peptide chain. The sequence is then repeated. An estimate of the rate of growth in this system is of a polypeptide chain lengthening by 40 amino acids per second.

2.6   Shall we not make another black box in which to lose ourselves?

The hypothesis linking therapies with a strong stress component in the change in the environment, and plastic adaptation of the neuromuscular system is not yet as clear as we would wish. But the credence given to the hypothesis by the exploration of the trophic code (cf. Chapter 7) is likely to become stronger as specific research into its full elucidation advances.

The greatest advances will be made if the laboratory-based workers (the technique freaks) start a meaningful dialogue with those of you at the sharp end of clinical rehabilitation. But let us avoid at all costs the making of a new black box (Fig. 2.9), where stress-rich therapies are employed carefully by you, with the effectiveness of the development of neuromuscular plasticity measured and assessed. But let it be a dialogue; the black box could otherwise become filled with neglected, modifiable molecules that seem to you to be just a little too unfamiliar: would not that be a terrible waste?

References

Cooper, J. R., Brown, F. E. and Roth, R. H. (1987) *Biochemical Basis of Neuropharmacology*. 5th edition. Oxford: Oxford University Press.

Shepherd, G. M. (1979) *The Synaptic Organization of the Brain*. Oxford: Oxford University Press.

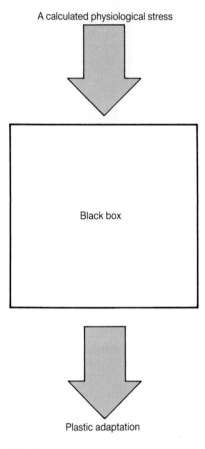

Fig. 2.9   Yet another black box, but we shall not let this one interfere with our professionalism, shall we? We will not ignore from now on its content of moveable molecules.

Shepherd, G. M. (1988) *Neurobiology*. Oxford: Oxford University Press.

Sherrington, C. S. (1906) *Integrative Action of the Nervous System*. New Haven: Yale University Press.

Chapter 3

Transmission of signals by neurons

3.1 A 'resting' potential? . . . surely not

There must be a reappraisal of the basic biophysical approach to nervous activity. Without intending any disrespect to the wealth of research into electrophysiology we intend to redress the balance towards the system that is a single neuron. An outline of the more important points in neurobiology has been presented clearly by Shepherd (1988).

Sherrington (1935) translated so well the writing of Ramón y Cajal where he described the application of silver staining to sections of the central nervous system (CNS) which had been fixed with potassium dichromate:

> Against a clear background stood black threadlets, some slender and smooth, some thick and thorny, in a pattern punctuated by small dense spots, stellate or fusiform. All was sharp as a sketch with Chinese ink on transparent Japan-paper.

That elegant technique in histology advanced the understanding of CNS structures, but it delayed an understanding of the true richness of nervous interaction in the brain. Some indication of the reason for that delay comes later in the translation:

> And to think that that was the same tissue which when stained with carmine or log-wood left the eye in a tangled thicket where sight may stare and grope forever fruitlessly.

We should attempt to build into our argument something which gives the solace of the early simplicity of the Golgi technique, as that neurohistology is named, but does not flinch from the shock of having to accept fully the complex interaction between neuron and environment in the sense of interaction which is employed in this book.

Living animal cells are bound by a plasma membrane and neurons are no exception. When the membrane is visualized at low power in an electron microscope it appears as a single dark line. With higher magnification it appears as two lines with a light space separating them. It will serve us best if we consider the plasma membrane as an interface between two differing and dilute solutions of electrolytes in water: one inside the neuron membrane (intracellular) and the other outside it (extracellular).

These two solutions differ from each other in their qualitative and quantitative characteristics. The molecular fragments obtained when sodium chloride dissolves in water are described as ions. The water separates and keeps the sodium ions from the chloride ions. The sodium ion yields an electron from its atom and so adopts a positive electric charge. The chloride atom receives this electron and takes to itself a negative electric charge. NaCl in dilute aqueous solution form Na^+ and Cl^- and just as nature abhors a vacuum, it is not overfond of ions left to their own devices.

A sphere is formed as water molecules surround and shield the effect of the exposed ions. Acting in this way the water molecules are dipoles (a separation of two equal, point electric charges of opposite sign by a small distance, Fig. 3.1). This occurs for all of the ions, for example, the two ionic species formed from NaCl are then said to be hydrated. To be a little more specific, the two ions are thought of as being surrounded by a hydrosphere of water molecules which gives them a definite hydrated radius.

The relative distribution of the ions of sodium (Na^+) and potassium (K^+) across the plasma membrane of a mammalian neuron can be illustrated diagrammatically as follows:

INSIDE	MEMBRANE	OUTSIDE
High [K$^+$]		Low [K$^+$]
Low [Na$^+$]		High [Na$^+$]

The convention of enclosing the symbol of the ion in square brackets, e.g. [Na$^+$], is read as: concentration of sodium ion.

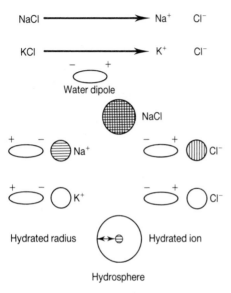

Fig. 3.1 When sodium chloride (NaCl) dissolves in water (H$_2$O), the water molecules allow the formation of negatively charged ions (anions) which are attracted towards, or are held by, a positive electric charge. Similarly, there are formed ions with a +ve electric charge (cations) attracted to, or held by, a −ve electric charge. Water molecules adopt a dipole form to permit this to happen. This form prevents, by its orientation, any neutralization of the electric charges on the sodium and chloride ions (Na$^+$ and Cl$^-$). A similar orientation is found with K$^+$ and Cl$^-$. The spherical orientation of the water dipoles leads to a hydrated ion and the formation of a hydrosphere with a definite radius of hydration.

The imbalance of ions across the plasma membrane is maintained by membrane pumps. These are energized by neuron metabolism which is coupled to them by **a**denosine **tri**phosphate (ATP). When molecules of ATP are hydrolysed to the diphosphate (ADP) the *energy* available as −P (high, applicable-energy phosphate bond) favours the transport of ions against their concentration gradient. They are, in other words, transported 'up-hill', and the membrane characteristics which allow and maintain this state are described by Fig. 3.2 (refer also once again to Fig. 1.1).

The word *pump* does no justice to the beauty of the membrane mechanism which must be close to the heart of life. A *pump* that is specific for Na$^+$ and K$^+$ is a (Na$^+$:K$^+$)–ATP*ase*. The suffix 'ase' is a conventional way of describing a molecule as an enzyme. The membrane pump is an enzyme which encourages the hydrolysis of ATP to ADP, so releasing usefully a chemical bond energy which powers the movement of ions in a direction against their concentration gradient (see above). The enzyme ATPase works effectively as an enzyme when K$^+$ is present in the extracellular fluid, or on the outside of the plasma membrane, and ATP and Na$^+$ are in the intracellular fluid, or on the inside of the plasma membrane. The interaction between the pump molecule and, alternately, the Na$^+$ and K$^+$, brings about allosteric changes in the molecule[1]. The allosteric changes transform the membrane molecule to an ion-transporting system. The enzyme which is required for catalysing the chemical reaction to hydrolyse ATP rapidly and easily, delivers −P to the pump, which requires for its own activity the Na$^+$ and K$^+$ to be located at sites within the intracellular and extracellular fluids from where they can be pumped 'uphill' in the stage of generation of the 'resting' electrical potential across the plasma membrane (it is an *electrogenic* pump).

The membrane pump is described sometimes as an antiport, because it transports across the membrane two different ions (Na$^+$ and K$^+$) in opposite directions. The diagram of Fig. 3.3 illustrates the action of an antiport.

Parts of a neuron membrane act passively, as though it were an electric cable. When the cable characteristics interact with active membrane macromolecules, the state of *available energy* inherent in those active patches of membrane give nerve its nervousness and neurons the ability to respond to stimuli by changes in excitability. This is the point where 'resting' potential should be redefined as a potential of preparedness for action. The maintenance of transmembrane potential by the pumping of ions during the times between action potentials requires the neuron to be in a state that is far from 'resting'. Similarly, the re-establishment of the ion gradients which follows the ion fluxes of the action potential also requires an application of metabolic energy coupled to the ion

---

[1] Allosteric can be translated as 'another form', and it refers here to the change in macromolecular form in a membrane that allows it to act as an ion pump

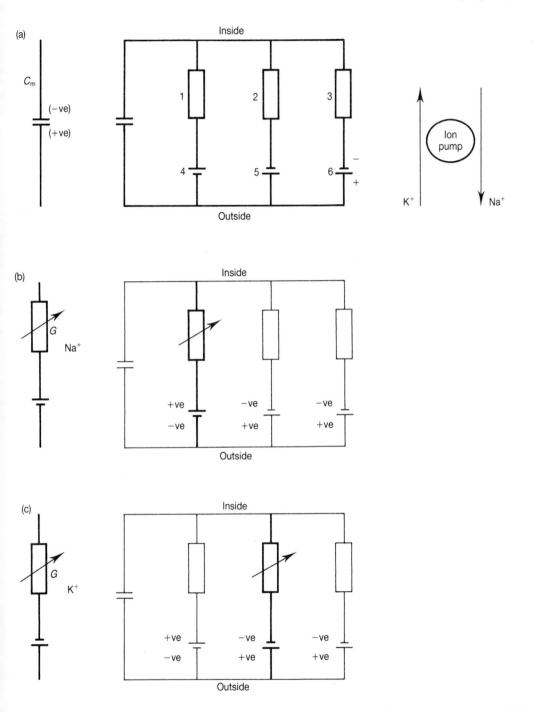

Fig. 3.2 (a) A simple diagram of the equivalent circuits of a neuron membrane. The electrical capacitance (C_m) keeps apart and holds the electric charge that is formed across it (polarization). An ion pump linked to the neuron metabolism is able to move Na$^+$ and K$^+$ in opposite directions and is able also to transport them against their concentration gradients. Circuit elements 4 and 5 are ion pumps for Na$^+$ and K$^+$, respectively. Element 6 is the electric potential which is able to direct leakage outflow of ions of $-$ve electric charge (e.g. Cl$^-$). (b) and (c) Rectangles 1, 2 and 3 are ion specific channels which allow ion conductivity changes (G_{Na+} and $G_K{}^+$) as a signal of an excitatory response by the neuron.

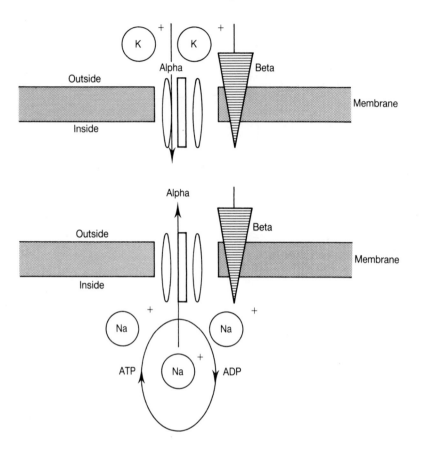

Fig. 3.3 A diagrammatic illustration of a membrane macromolecule acting as an ion pump. The alpha-unit of the protein acts as an ATPase. The beta-unit, a glycoprotein, is incompletely understood. Conformational changes of the alpha-unit of the protein acts as a contrapump moving Na^+ and K^+ ions across the membrane against their respective concentration gradients. In the two diagrams, the pumping actions are shown as being separate. They are in fact one. This presentation is to ease understanding. Refer once again to the text of Chapter 3 and to Chapter 1, Section 1.1.

pumps. The proportion of the total neuron metabolism involved in the maintenance of the 'resting' potential is approximately 30% but this rises to 75% during the phase of restoration of the internal $[Na^+]$ following the 'dam-burst' influx during the rising phase of the action potential when Na^+ conductance by ion channels (see below) is increased.

The sensitivity of the ATPase to the intracellular $[Na^+]$ is a remarkable way of restoring the balance of Na^+ across the neuronal membrane so as to maintain a stable threshold of excitation for the neuron in the face of the generation of trains of action potentials. In addition to our reappraisal of the term 'resting' potential it would be better to put 'action' in inverted commas also to remind us that the concentration differences maintained by the ion pumps across the neuronal membrane ensure a 'preparedness' for action. The increases of Na^+ and K^+ conductances are responsible respectively for the rising limb of the action potential and the beginning of the phase of membrane recovery as the 'preparedness' potential is restored ready for

another cycle of ion flow. The neuron, in preparation for this, detects, measures and calculates the significance of the amount of excitation/inhibition it is receiving at the synapses on the soma and dendritic surface (see Chapter 4).

The neuron membrane is an array of the equivalent circuits illustrated in Fig. 3.2a. In the simplest terms, the membrane can be considered as as electrical capacitor which holds the charge of the 'resting' membrane potential, the passive physical characteristics of which should be considered as a high physical resistance separating two liquids of lower physical resistance: these are the intracellular and extracellular fluid phases. Figure 3.2 includes an element of membrane capacitance which stores the electric charge across the neuronal membrane. It is the time course of the depolarization of this element of capacitance (a capacitor) that provides the neuron with a real threshold which must be reached before the neuron can signal by the discharge of an action potential. The event signalled by the propagation of an action potential is that

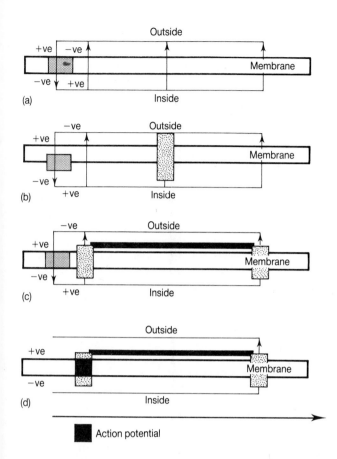

Fig. 3.4 (a) When a patch of axon membrane has its 'resting' potential artificially reversed (stippled rectangle) a passive current flow is established. This current runs from inside to outside of the axon. (b) Should the current flow encounter a patch of ion conductance channels (heavily stippled rectangle) an action potential will be generated. (c) When the patches of conductance are separated by a sheath of myelin (heavy line), the generation of an action potential cannot occur except at the nodes of Ranvier. (d) Replacing the artificial reversal of membrane potential by an action potential shows the myelin to have a similar restriction on the propagation of an action potential.

a meaningful resultant of excitation/inhibition has been calculated from the excitatory- (E-) and inhibitory- (I-) postsynaptic potentials (PSPs) (see also Chapter 4).

With reference, for a moment, to Fig. 3.4a we see that if the 'resting' membrane potential is artificially and locally reversed (indicated by a localized heavy stippling) from inside −ve and outside +ve states to a state where the inside is +ve and the outside −ve, an electric circuit is established which involves a length of membrane. This is a passive phenomenon which assumes nothing more than that the neuron membrane acts as an electric cable with any leakage of electrical current limited by its highly resistive elements.

The ion pumps, which are polypeptide molecules as membrane components, are specific for transporting different species of ion, for example, ions 1, 2 and 3 in Fig. 3.2a. If these were capable of acting independently, they would contribute charge to the membrane with the polarities shown in Fig. 3.2b (4, 5 and 6). Wherever the passive flow of current across the neuron membrane encounters one of these membrane modules, there is a change from passive to active characteristics.

The rectangles 1, 2 and 3 represent active, conductance channels for the ions shown to the left of Fig. 3.2b and c. Conductance may not be familiar to you, in which case it can be defined as:

$$\text{Conductance} = 1/\text{Resistance}$$

So, whereas passive cable characteristics of the neuronal membrane depend upon a high membrane resistance, the involvement of the membrane in activity is just the reverse. It involves then a system of current carrying or conductance by the transport of the electric charge of the several forms of ion flowing.

The Na^+:K^+ ion pumps are, in fact, macromolecules as membrane components. It is difficult to see how molecules, which we comprehend usually as 'chemistry', can be so effective in generating electric potentials and current flow, which we comprehend with equivalent determination as 'physics'.

There is only one piece of advice we can offer to those of you who, very sensibly, shirk from thinking of life as improbability and order as negative entropy (negentropy). It is this: hang in there. If it is of any consolation to you, a spouse amongst us has a clear idea of the definition of the ultimate disorder of entropy. It is the drawer in which one's socks are kept.

When the state of an ion channel in part of the neuron membrane is sensitive to the voltage across it, it is described as a voltage-dependent or a voltage-gated channel. When it is sensitive to a neurotransmitter, released, for example, at a synapse, it is described as a transmitter-dependent channel (see Chapter 4). In one mode of action, therefore, ion channels formed by macromolecules permit ions to pass through them according to the electric potential difference across the membrane. At one time, this characteristic distinguished impulse channels involved in signal propagation from synaptic channels which were presumed to be sensitive only to the action of neurotransmitter molecules. It is believed now, however, that voltage-dependent channels can be sensitive also to neurotransmitter molecules. Demonstrations of such voltage-dependent, synaptic channels have been made on cell cultures made from dorsal root ganglia (Dunlap and Fischbach, 1978).

The density of occurrence of voltage-gated channels varies greatly over the membrane surface of a neuron. Referring once again to Fig. 3.4 we see in part b one example of a series of voltage-sensitive patches illustrated by the rectangle of heavy stippling. Whenever the passive current flow is intercepted by such a locus of patches, a regenerative region of membrane 'boosts' the current flow by the generation of a new action potential. The passive flow of current resulting from this action potential repeats the series – passive current flow and a response of another regenerative region. This smooth transmission of an action potential is typical of the non-myelinated axonal processes of some neurons.

The passive flow of current and its interaction with regenerative patches of membrane makes us realize that the passive current flows in a volume of conductor (this is sometimes known as electrotonus) which is not as limited as Fig. 3.4 suggests. Important passive flows of electric current are generated by localized synaptic action on the dendritic branches of a neuron. When the direction of passive current flow involves the axon hillock of the neuron,

it begins to integrate the sum of excitation/inhibition taking place over the neuron soma and dendrite surface. If the resulting depolarization of the hillock reaches a threshold value, an action potential is generated and has two effects. The first is to propagate action potentials by regenerative saltation along the peripheral length of the axon, and the second is to invade the soma of the neuron and its dendritic array to a variable extent. This soma and dendritic potential makes the flow of passive current around the neuron body extremely complex. It makes also the generation of action potential codes in the form of a train of impulses difficult to predict. One generator zone, for example, at the hillock of a motoneuron in the spinal cord, is just about understandable. Should 'hot spots' develop locally in the dendritic array of a neuron (Fig. 3.5), possibly as a stage of plastic adaptation, they would generate action potentials ectopically and locally as they sample the passive flow of dendritic current. The resulting variability of neuron integration of dendritic synaptic activity would add to the modes with which a neuron signals its involvement in the control systems of the CNS. Purkinje neurons of the mammalian cerebellar cortex are believed to behave in this manner.

By comparison with the frequently occurring regenerative patches in non-myelinated axons (see Fig. 3.4b) the presence of the wrapping of the axonal process by Schwann cell membrane (myelinization) concentrates the regenerative patches to

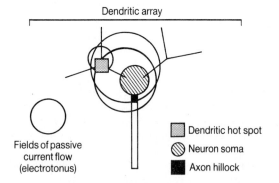

Fig. 3.5 The axon hillock of a neuron samples the field of passive current flow generated by synaptic activity on neuron soma and dendritic array. Trains of action potentials usually originate at the axon hillock. Dendritic 'hot-spots' can be formed also and they themselves contribute a localized and accessory action potential generator which adds to the richness of the fields of passive current flow. It contributes additionally to the pattern of action potentials propagated by the neuron.

the nodes of Ranvier along the length of an axon. It is possible that the presence of the Schwann cell over the internodal extent of the axon (Fig. 3.4c) both prevents the location of active membrane patches and encourages their localization in the nodes of Ranvier. At the nodes, the passive flow of current is most likely to operate a series of voltage-gated ion channels (Fig. 3.4c).

It has been said (Bishop, 1971) that the feudal services to a lord by his vassal were recorded as being 'the offering of: *unum saltum et siffletum et unum bumbulum*'. A partial translation of which gives us 'A leap and a whistle and . . .' with the remainder left untranslated and appropriately in the Middle Ages.

With the regenerative patches of axonal membrane localized to the infrequently occurring nodes of Ranvier, propagation of the action potential is described as *saltatory* because it leaps along the axonal length from one such localization to another.

3.2 Never mind the potential, feel the current

We should point out once more that there has been a shift in balance of emphasis in the academic subjects which relate to clinical rehabilitation. These are summarized again, this time as Fig. 3.6: anatomy and physiology have changed to the bioch*em*istry of macromolecules, where in the *e*lectron *m*icroscope the truth about rehabilitation is revealed. A general approach has grown in the last 30 years which on the one hand has united the basic medical sciences, but on the other has isolated them by reaction from those professionals with a more traditional approach to their subjects.

Neurochemistry is a young discipline, the validity of which was questioned until recently. Now, there is recognition of the unifying nature of biochemistry devoted to the nervous system within the more general molecular neurobiology. An outline of this modern approach to conventional neuroanatomy and neurophysiology is offered by Guroff (1980).

The signal that we thought of first as we planned this chapter was the action potential of the neuron. But *one* all-or-nothing response of a neuron to threshold excitation is an oversimplification. When we consider instead the distance over which trains of the signal have to be propagated, time after time after time, we come to realize that it is the mainten-

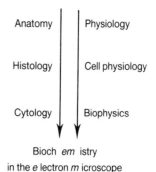

Bioch *em* istry
in the *e* lectron *m* icroscope
you can see the anatomy of the biochemistry doing the physiology

Fig. 3.6 The disciplines of basic medical science have changed, and in doing so they have become more relevant to rehabilitation. Two evolving lines move from anatomy and physiology to unite in bioch*em*istry. We owe the statement of unity to the late Dr T. G. Richards.

ance of the structural integrity of the propagating system that is of prime importance.

The neuron must not be thought of as a structure, without internal variability, which exists only to signal to other cells: this means both neuron-to-neuronal, and neuronal-to-muscular. We are limiting ourselves by assuming that this occurs solely by the generation, propagation and transmission of action potentials. It was when neurons were studied by conventional microscopy, following staining with metallic salts or dyes, that the idea of the immutability of neurons took root in the minds of histologists. The size and clarity of single neuron action potentials took a different hold on the minds of those electrophysiologists who employed microelectrodes or intracellular pipettes to isolate electrically *the small still voice* of single neurons from the *noise* of surrounding cells.

A breakthrough in this battle for minds came at the time when the microscopic image of a living neuron could be recorded by a video camera. Digitization of the image from the camera followed, and when the digital image was fed to a computer it could be enhanced and displayed in various ways. The resulting visualization of the ceaseless movement of cell particles along the microtubular structures within the neuron, particularly along its axonal process, resolved into a bidirectional transport systen. It is believed now that this axonal transport has an essential part to play in the maintenance of the structural integrity of the cell. It has, additionally, a part to play in the plastic adaptation of the neuron.

Recollection of early arguments between schools of neurophysiology recalls the '*soup or spark*' controversy which raged over whether or not synaptic transmission was due simply to a modification in effectiveness of local circuits of electrical flow (*spark*), or if an intermediate step was introduced involving synthesis, storage and release of a *soup* of neurotransmitter molecules: the *soup* hypothesis prevailed (see Chapter 4).

It is worth remembering that the rate of natural, developmental growth and the rate of regenerative axonal growth that follows peripheral nerve transection corresponds to the slower rate at which intracellular materials are transported by axonal flow (1–2 mm a day; see Table 3.1). We should not separate completely, therefore, the two components of the system of neuronal signalling. But, until a causal relationship can be shown to exist between the two forms of neuronal signalling: the transmission of a membrane signal (the wave of ionic permeability change across the neuron membrane) and the systems of axonal transport, we have to accept that the relationship is only casual. We should recognize that a firmly established link between the two modes of signalling by neurons is yet to be found.

Table 3.1 Axonal transport.

Type of transport	Velocity of transport	Materials transported
I	240 mm/day	Membrane protein components
II	75.0–78.0 mm/day	Mitochondria
III	5.0–10.0 mm/day	Myosins
IV	2.0–5.0 mm/day	Tubulins, myocin actin
V	0.7–1.0 mm/day	Neurofilament protein

Adapted from Guroff (1980)

The possibility of an axon 'time sharing' with two different systems of information transfer is attractive, and one example is discussed below in Chapter 7, Section 7.6. The possibility of 'time sharing' discussed there involves the simultaneous transmission of two trains of action potentials over a single axon. One of the trains involves in action immediately a part of the central nervous system as the train finds it. Whereas the other directs and controls the eventual plastic adaptation of the CNS to meet better the requirements for behavioural change. We should draw attention to a further point with regard to the separation of the signals

of excitation from those of the nutritional or trophic influences that a neuron might have on muscle or a neuron might have upon another neuron. These are discussed elsewhere (Gutmann, 1969; see also Chapter 7, Section 7.7).

3.3   Non-impulse neurons

We do not know whether or not we have succeeded in introducing to you the concept of 'time sharing' in the nervous system with any degree of success (cf. Chapter 3, Section 3.2). If we have not there will be another attempt made in Chapter 7, Section 7.7. This may not be a suitable time therefore to introduce the thought of neurons which do not have axons which fit either of the 'longer-than-dendrites' or possessing 'the hot-spot of the axon hillock' models.

Table 3.2 First and second messenger molecules and their reception by the growth cone. The order is alphabetic and does not suggest any order of importance to the system.

Messenger	Role
Ca+ (2nd)	Actin/myosin interaction, CANPs
cAMP (2nd)	
DA dopamine (1st)	Transmitter in dopaminergic pathways
GABA (1st)	Inhibitory transmitter
GP glycoprotein	Membrane component
5-Hydroxy tryptamine (5HT)	(1st, or precursor)
Nor-adrenalin (NA) (1st)	Transmitter, hormone
Substance P (SP) (1st)	Transmitter
NCAM	Transmitter in the axon reflex Neuron cell adhesion molecule
Neuron-glia cell adhesion molecule (NG-CPM)	Membrane component
Protease (2nd)	
Vasoactive intentinal peptide (VIP) (1st,2nd?)	

At worst we are anticipating Chapter 4, so we will give the concept a whirl. We have introduced the idea of local and graded, non-propagated electrical responses. They do not signal action by the *bravura* assembly of a train of spike potentials each with an all-or-nothing characteristic. That sort of signalling is fine when projection of what is being signalled has to travel long distances in the body (e.g. by means of the spinal motoneuron in humans).

Signalling is very much faster if the consequence of excitation in the nervous system is signalled by the setting up of a field of potential. In the generation of action potentials travelling over an axon, each potential is repeatedly set up, or regenerated, at every 'hot-spot' encountered at the nodes of Ranvier of that axon. The action currents (cf. Fig. 3.4) travel further than the next node of Ranvier but, because the sensitivity of that 'hot spot' is so great, it makes the current flow redundant as it fires its own action potential. The 'setting-up-time' for each action potential in a train takes much longer than the series of nudges that ion gives to ion in aqueous solution during the electronic signalling as action current is generated.

Neurons with very short or no axons (anaxonic neurons or amacrine neurons) transfer information to other neurons in analogue as opposed to digital codes. A digital signal requires pulse intervals to convey information (e.g. the on–off activity of codes in a digital computer). The digital computer is said to be 'thick' but each 'thick' decision is made quickly. An analogue computer is able to handle information just as quickly as it chooses to sample a signal of an infinitely variable amplitude (none of your all-or-nothing stuff here please). An axonal neuron requires only to have a suitably responsive membrane molecule within reach. There is a neurophysiology of this form of analogue which can be found in the CNS but we do not have enough space here to treat it with respect. We do recommend the development of this subject as it is given by Shepherd (1981, 1988).

3.4 The growth cone as a signal receiver

The molecular neurobiology of the growth cone, the structure formed at the exploring end of developing or repairing axons or dendrites, will be discussed fully in Chapter 8. We must introduce here though a brief introduction to the neurite, and the molecular signals it receives (see Table 3.2).

The name neurite can mean *all things to all men*. It can be employed ambiguously as a cell process. The name is limited sometimes to the dendritic processes of invertebrates, but within the context of this book we will ask you to accept its definition as 'a process of a mammalian neuron in a stage of development, of growth or of repair when the nature of the eventual process is uncertain because it is still immature'. It is, to be more straightfor-

ward, a sprout or shoot issuing from an exploring neuron.

The growth cone is dirigible. It is amoeboid in character and is directed towards the goal which requires it as it 'tastes' its way through its complex chemical environment. Ramón y Cajal with his remarkable foresight chose the appropriate material to study and drew from his studies the correct conclusions concerning his results (cf. Sherrington, 1935). The process of growth cone function, although Cajal was undoubtedly correct, requires additionally the facility of recognition of the appropriate cell and the ability to adhere to it once it is recognized.

This point in the argument concerning nervous function recalls the 'soup or spark' arguments, which now seem so long ago. It appears to be the watershed of neuroscience. On the one hand there is the molecular 'soup' and on the other we have as we mentioned the *bravura* construction of trains of action potentials: the 'sparks'. It is a matter of 'you pays your money and you takes your pick'. It will be the acid test of the successfulness of this book: the ability to understand the time-sharing of dissimilar signals from the two systems of information transfer we have at our fingertips. Something keeps running through the writer's mind: '*how happy would I be with either, were t'other fair charmer away*'.

We must now refute the arguments of those who deny, most obdurately, the existence of neuromuscular plasticity. New neurons (with the exception of the few cited above) cannot be generated in the postnatal nervous system. Each mature neuron however retains not only the ability to form new neuronal processes and synapses, it feels a pressure to do so. It has been said that 'whereas all animals have an urge to live, humans alone have a zest for life'. If the cells of the neuromuscular system were 'hard-wired', and even if the circuitry of wiring was as elaborate as that of the most powerful computer known, we should be unable to learn new skills as we do learn them, remember them as we do remember them, and continuously and progressively improve upon the skills we are learning.

All of the *urge* and at least a small part of the *zest* appears as the primer in the cell nuclei of nerve and muscle. This appears to demand new connections and the development of a new effectiveness of action where the orginal has been lost. It is almost as though neurons, to take one example, *know* of the details of connectivity which were needed once to carry out a nervous control, and details needed still to re-establish new controls. These can then guide rehabilitation, by trophicity, along a path towards its own maturation (see Chapter 7).

How inadequate and imprecise human language is when it attempts to comment on the communication between the cells of the neuromuscular system. A full discussion of signalling by neurons will have to be approached again (Chapter 6) and yet again (Chapter 9) before we can attempt to describe the marvels of the 'tapestry' of rehabilitation (Affeldt, 1988).

References

Affeldt, J. E. (1988) The tapestry of rehabilitation, its weavers and its threads. *J. Allied Health* **2**; 53–58.

Bishop, M. (1971) *The Penguin Book of the Middle Ages.* Harmondsworth: Penguin Books.

Cottrell, G. A. and Usherwood, P. N. R. (1973) *Synapses* Proceedings of the International Symposium. Scottish Electrophysiological Society. Volume 29. Glasgow: Blackie.

Dunlap, K. and Fischbach, G. D. (1978) Neurotransmitters decrease calcium component of sensory neuron potentials. *Nature* **276**: 137–9.

Morrison, A. R. and Strick, P. L. (1982) *Changing Concepts of the Nervous System.* London: Academic Press.

Guroff, G. (1980 *Molecular Neurobiology.* New York: Dekker.

Gutmann, E. (1969) The trophic function of the nerve cell. *Scientia* **194**; 1–20.

Hodgkin, A. L. (1964) *The Conduction of the Nervous Impulse. Sherrington Lecture VII.* Liverpool: The University Press.

Katz, B. (1966) *Nerve, Muscle and Synapse.* New York: McGraw Hill, Inc.

Roberts, A. and Bush, B. M. H. eds. (1981) *Without Impulses.* Cambridge: Cambridge University Press.

Shepherd, G. M. (1981) The nerve impulse and the nature of nervous function. In: Roberts, A. and Bush, B. M. H. eds. *Without Impulses.* Cambridge: Cambridge University Press, pp. 1–27.

Shepherd, G. M. (1988) *Neurobiology.* Oxford: Oxford University Press.

Sherrington, C. S. (1935) Santiago Ramón y Cajal 1852–1934. *Obituary Notices of the Royal Society of London* **4**: 425–41.

Chapter 4

Synaptic transmission

4.1 Review of the propagation of action potentials over axons

Non-myelinated axons were described as using cable conduction (cf. the Glossary) to transfer excitation along the neuron from the point of reception of the stimulus to the next excitable neuron or to another effector structure. This is illustrated in Fig. 4.1.

The cable properties of an axon are poor when compared with the conducting properties of a metal cable. The poor cable conductance of a non-myelinated axon is improved by a 'booster' (see Chapter 3) linked to the bioenergetic system of the neuron. Without such a booster, the action potential would be reduced in amplitude as it passed over the length of the axon. In other words, the signal would become distorted or suffer decrement during its propagation. This is prevented by localizations within the axon membrane of patches of self-regenerating sodium conductance (the outside-to-inside flow of the sodium ion Na^+). These are distributed along the entire length of the axon from the point of excitation of the axon to the point of its effect.

In spite of metabolic boosters, cable conduction is relatively slow in the non-myelinated axon (Table 4.1).

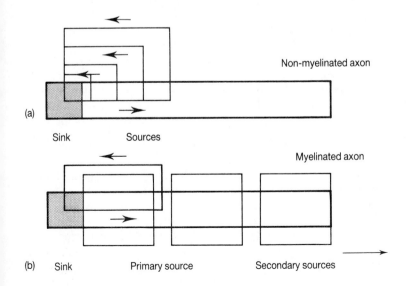

Non-myelinated axon

(a)

Sink   Sources

Myelinated axon

(b)   Sink   Primary source   Secondary sources

Fig. 4.1 A simplified diagram of the cable characteristics in (a) a non-myelinated axon, and (b) a myelinated axon. The excited region of an axon (shaded) acts as a 'sink; into which current flows from 'sources' in the unexcited membrane. When the flow of current from a 'source' approaches threshold, the 'source' generates a newly excited area of membrane. The expression 'action current' is preferable therefore to action potential. (a) In non-myelinated axons 'booster' regions (see text) are evenly distributed and not restricted by the presence of Schwann cells. (b) In myelinated axons the electrical characteristics of the Schwann cell population along its length restricts effective current flow to 'sources' and 'sinks' limited to the membrane exposed at the nodes of Ranvier.

Table 4.1 Classification of axons.

Axon type	Axon function	Average axon diameter (μ)m	Average conduction velocity (ms^{-1})
A-alpha	Primary muscle spindle afferents	15	100
A-alpha	Motor to skeletal muscle	9	50
A-beta	Fusimotor–skeletomotor	7	20
A-beta	Cutaneous touch and pressure	8	20
A-gamma	Fusimotor	5	20
A-delta	Cutaneous temperature and pain afferents	3	15
B	Sympathetic preganglionic	3	13
C	**Sympathetic postganglionic**	**1**	**1**
	Pain afferents	**<1**	**<1**

Bold print: non-myelinated.

Myelinated and non-myelinated are unfortunate adjectives. Both types of axon are associated structurally with glial cells which align themselves longitudinally along the developing axon. If the axons develop as non-myelinated, several of them share the envelopment of the glial cells aligned along their length.

With a peripheral axon determined as myelinated, specialized glial cell (Schwann or satellite cells) change with respect to their longitudinal alignment with a single axon, and appear to wrap it in numerous layers of their own cell membrane.

This lipid–protein sheath has a very low proportion of protein to lipid and acts, in part, as an insulator preventing the flow of electric current across the axonal membrane. The sheath formed by the Schwann cells acts to reduce also the electrical capacitance between the axon cylinder and the surrounding extracellular fluid. This means that much less of the inward current is lost by electric shunting.

4.2 Propagation: conduction compared with transmission

Both examples of propagation of an action potential discussed so far have been initiated by a flow of current between an activated (excited) and an unactivated (unexcited) region of an axon. Imagine a wall, or more exactly, a membrane septum interrupting the continuity of the axon cylinder (Fig. 4.2). Further imagine a gap or cleft being formed

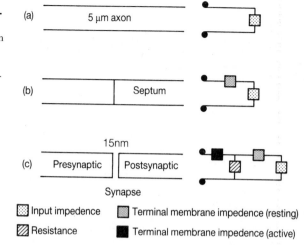

Fig. 4.2 Cable characteristics of an axon can be applied only to the most simple situations. (a) A small diameter non-myelinated axon adds only an impedence characteristic to transmission. (b) Should the continuity of the cable be interrupted by a septum a second element of impedence is introduced. (c) When a synaptic cleft is also introduced, the number of both resistive and impedance elements is increased. This argues that when transmission is compared with propagation, something other than electrical, cable transmission must be introduced. This is the presynaptic release of transmitter molecules and the reaction of them with molecular receptors in the postsynaptic membrane. Definitions: Full definition of terms, which could be unfamiliar to you, will be found in the Glossary.

by two membranes (a cleft, for example, 15 nm wide) in the cable conduction line of an axon. We will consider two forms of such a junction. The axon and its possible synaptic connections will have to be thought of as being biophysical, with the neuron involved in a controlled and variable biosythesis of those macromolecules which contribute to the physical properties of the cell. Details of the electric characteristics involved in this comparison between propagation and transmission may be omitted during a first reading of this chapter. When it becomes clear to you that the detail cannot be ignored if a full understanding of plasticity is to be obtained, it will be found in the Appendix.

The simplest form of synapse is the nerve–muscle junction (motor endplate or neuromuscular synapse). This operates as a simple relay at which a nerve impulse is transmitted with a high factor of safety and with minimum delay from the motoneuron axon to a large number of muscle fibres. The number of muscle fibres innervated by the branches of a single motoneuron axon is expressed as the innervation ratio.

The motoneuron, its axon and branches with all of the muscle fibres they innervate (the muscle unit), are together called the motor unit. Sherrington (1906) referred to this unit as the 'final common path' of the motor system. Once the decision that the force is to be generated by a motor unit is taken by the motoneuron pools of the spinal cord or brain stem, it has to be applied in a controlled movement. To defend the force available to a discharging motoneuron, the endplate can undergo a form of plastic adaptation. The adaptation involves sprouting of the axon terminal, usually at a node of Ranvier immediately proximal to the terminal of the sprouting axon. This results in rejuvenation of the endplate, with the original endplate degenerating prior to resorption. Similar sprouting can yield substitution of an endplate (Tuffery, 1971).

The argument emerging gradually from this discussion of transmission across the neuromuscular synapse returns us to the inescapable. When considering the maintenance influence on (skeletal) muscle mediated by the nerve a multiple control of maintenance must be assumed (Gutmann, 1969). A clear development of the multiple controls and their expression as neuromuscular plasticity and trophic effects is presented by Morrison and Strick (1982).

A discussion of the release of non-transmitter substances at the neuromuscular synapse (Vrbová *et al.*, 1978) introduces us to the transmission not only of action currents and their consequences at the synapse but also through the agency of an interaction of neurotransmitter molecules and the postsynaptic molecular receptors together with transmission of information required for the neuromuscular system to undergo a purposeful plastic adaptation. Vrbová (1989) describes a co-release of acetylcholine molecules and 'trophic molecules' into the synaptic cleft of the neuromuscular junction. Vrbová (1989) describes additionally the provision of an endocrine profile of hormones acting in association with other substances to enable a full muscular response in plastic adaptation. These will be referred to further in Chapter 7.

The second form, the nerve–nerve junction (neuronal synapse), again transmits an impulse or more exactly a pattern of impulses, but in doing so it transcribes them into graded and localized subthreshold potential at the postsynaptic membrane (Fig. 4.3).

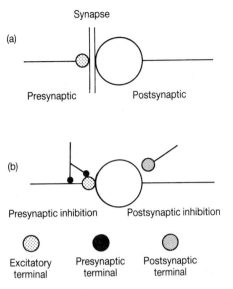

Fig. 4.3 The synapse is a gap in the conduction system. On first analysis it is better to describe what it is that precedes it (presynaptic) and what comes after it (postsynaptic). (a) The presynaptic element (hatched circle) has activity controlled by, and metabolism determined by, the presynaptic neuron and its nucleus, respectively. (b) Presynaptic inhibition is not applied to the postsynaptic neuron membrane, but to the membrane of the presynaptic element. It acts not by modifying the membrane potential of the postsynaptic neuron, but by reducing the quantity of transmitter molecules released into the synaptic cleft. The key to the terminals is shown at the bottom of the figure.

4.3 Presynaptic and postsynaptic

The parts of a neuron membrane defined as being before (presynaptically) and after (postsynaptically) the cleft of the synapse are the best way of separating, in discussion, these two elements of the vertebrate central nervous system (CNS) structure. The presynaptic membrane of the synapse is a part of the presynaptic axon. It is a flattened point of contact of a single, synaptic ending with the postsynaptic surface on the next neuron in the chain.

We discussed the method of propagation (Chapter 3) in both non-myelinated and in myelinated axons. We described also how the axon current generated by the action potential suffered no decrement as it was transmitted over the axon length. A different although no less effective mechanism is found when the action potential is transmitted across the junction of the synapse. This situation, which requires more than a simple description, is found when an axon either branches or tapers: this was discussed with respect to regeneration in dendritic branches (Chapter 3).

The action potential is propagated into the terminal, whereupon its activity as an electrical event ends. The action current it generates before it does so is responsible for the release of neurotransmitter into the synaptic cleft. Before its release, the neurotransmitter is stored in vesicles contained in the synaptic ending. They are then released and the neurotransmitter diffuses to transmitter receptor molecules which form a component of the postsynaptic membrane.

The binding of receptor molecule and molecular receptor in the membrane has two possible effects. The first is that of opening channels able to conduct a flow (a flux) of specific ions: these are referred to as iontophores. The second is the release from its site in the neuron membrane of a G-protein system (this was introduced in Chapters 1 and 2). The flow through iontophores contributes to the generation of a new action potential in the postsynaptic element of the neuronal chain. The G-protein system is active during plastic adaptation, and is discussed again in that special context in Chapters 1 and 7.

The neurotransmitter bound to the receptor molecule is split by an appropriate enzyme. The transmitter acetylcholine, to give one example, is split by the enzyme acetylcholine esterase. The separate acetyl ions and choline ions can then be reabsorbed by the synaptic terminal. After resynthesis, aided by the enzyme acetylcholine acetylase, the molecules are utilized as neurotransmitter and are again released by action potentials during subsequent activity.

4.4   Snapshot or cine-film?

The preceding and elementary description of synaptic transmission gives a *static* picture: a snap-shot of the events involved. A more *dynamic* picture, a cine-film, for example, must be obtained if we are to understand the adaptation of those events at synapses which are revealed by variation of synaptic transmission. The stages involved in the propagation and transmission of action potentials, along an axon and across a synapse, can be shown as a series of discrete steps (Fig. 4.4).

Each step must be reconsidered from the point of view of them taking place at a molecular level; not as a simple description of the macromolecules

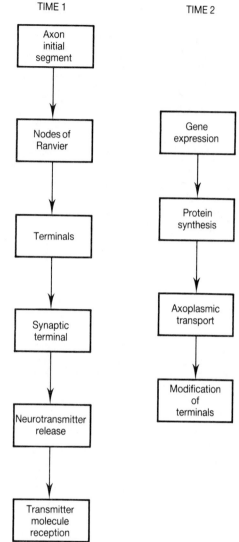

Fig. 4.4   A simple description of the propagation of an action potential and its transmission across a synapse deals with time in the simplest of approaches. That time (TIME 1) will explain such parameters as the latency of a response following a stimulus. It will allow also a calculation of conduction velocity. To understand the time course leading to plastic adaptation (TIME 2) allows a description of the course of events leading from a significant change in environment of the neuron acting through modified gene expression. TIME 2 takes into account also the process of axoplasmic transport and molecular insertion or replacement in the membrane.

involved (Chapters 1 and 2), but a description of the dynamics of those macromolecules: what it is that stimulates their formation, the site of their for-

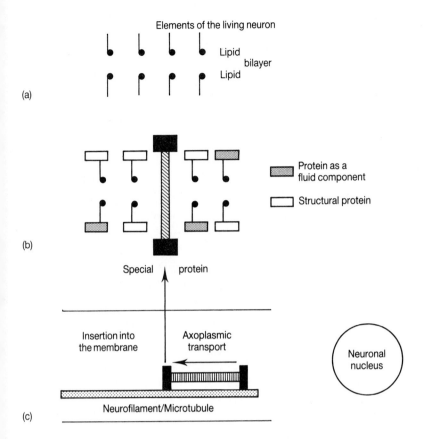

Elements of the living neuron

(a)

Lipid
bilayer
Lipid

(b)

Protein as a
fluid component

Structural protein

Special   protein

Insertion into
the membrane

Axoplasmic
transport

Neuronal
nucleus

Neurofilament/Microtubule

(c)

Fig. 4.5 A schematic illustration of the basic structural molecular components of a membrane. (a) The lipid–lipid molecules form what is known as a bilayer. Think of the membrane as being fluid, in part stabilized by a few structural protein molecules but allowing special proteins synthesized in the neuron soma and transported by the neurofilament and microtubule structures which are involved in axoplasmic transport (c). (b) The special protein can be inserted into the fluid membrane to replace or complement other proteins.

mation, their transport after formation and their location in the excitable membrane.

4.5 Membrane signalling and axonal (or axoplasmic) transport

It may seem strange to be asked to accept that the propagation and transmission of action potentials over the membrane of a neuronal system are only two of its activities. The all-or-nothing nature of the action potential should tell us that it is a very limited way of transmitting a flow of information through a system: particularly in a system that shows plastic adaptation. You will recall the definition (Brown and Hardman, 1987, in Winlow and McCrohan, 1987, and cited in the Introduction) of plasticity as '. . . the ability of cells to alter any aspect of their phenotype . . . in response to abnormal changes in their state or environment'.

We must now turn to a discussion of the second form of flow (cf. Chapter 3 and Table 3.1), the flow

of molecules which takes place through the internal structures of the neuron. These are the soma of the neuron, the cylinder of its axon and the branching and tapering, hollow system of its dendrites. The flow of information comprises transport systems of the axoplasm, or its equivalent in soma and dendrites. Examples of substances transported are, in ascending order of size: precursor molecules from which neurotransmitter molecules are synthesized, macromolecules to be used as membrane components and mitochondria to provide energy for synthetic reactions in structures (e.g. synaptic endings) peripheral to the neuron soma.

This concept of material transport in nerve, together with the part it plays in the development of the nervous system, the maintenance of that effective development and during its repair after injury or disease are summarized clearly by Ochs (1974) and will not be repeated here. A simple diagram will introduce those points relevant to our discussion (Fig. 4.5).

4.6 Dynamic equilibrium of synaptic structures

The simplest form of equilibrium in the molecular components of a synapse is shown in Fig. 4.6a where molecules have a lifetime of stability. A much more exact form of equilibrium is one where the molecules broken down by catabolism are replaced by a synthesis during anabolism. This form would give a dynamic equilibrium (Fig. 4.6b). Admitting plasticity to our arguments, a molecule catabolized would be replaced by a directed anabolism providing the neuron with molecules more suitable for a required adaptation. This is shown in Fig. 4.6c. Catabolism together with a related anabolism are sometimes referred to collectively as metabolism. We feel that the duality used here leads us to see more clearly the dynamics of the process and the complexity within which it operates. More importantly, it suggests that plastic adaptation can be predicted and controlled.

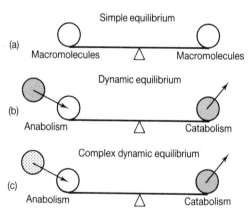

Fig. 4.6 (a) Special protein molecules associated with membrane activity are seldom in a simple equilibrium. (b) The basis of plastic adaptation is where those molecules are in a dynamic equilibrium and molecular breakdown (catabolism) is balanced by protein synthesis (anabolism) of an identical protein at a rate which balances its breakdown. (c) Plastic adaptation shows a full adaptive response when a molecule is anabolized under the control of gene expression responding to an effective change in neuronal environment.

4.7 Excitation and inhibition at synapses

Section 4.2 was concerned with synaptic transmission, and with making a comparison of it with the propagation of a wave of excitation travelling over an axon. It was reasonable therefore to discuss excitatory synapses only. In the neuromuscular synapse (the endplate) in vertebrates excitation only is present. When we turn to consider inhibition together with excitation and further develop the integration of the two activities we should remember the following statement:

> Desistence from action may be as truly active as the taking of action. In the animal organism, side by side with excitation to action run restraints from action. Only recently has account been taken of the frequency of occurrence of this restraint and of the fact that restraint by inhibition is as fully a reaction to the stimulus as is the excitatory response itself.
>
> Sherrington (1913)

4.8 The inhibitory synapse

The major differences between an excitatory and an inhibitory synapse can be found in the different area of contact an inhibitory synaptic terminal makes with the surface of the next neuron and then in the different transmitter molecule employed in an inhibitory synapse: gamma-aminobutryic acid by comparison with acetylcholine employed during excitation. The vesicles in which the two different transmitters are stored in the synaptic terminal are also of different shape.

> Synaptic vesicles like chocolates come in a variety of shapes and sizes, and are stuffed with different kinds of filling.
>
> Sanford Palay in Bloom and Fawcett (1975)

Plasticity of the neuromuscular system appearing as 'synaptic strengthening' and 'synaptic sprouting' will be discussed in Chapter 4 and, in preparation for this, we will present here a transition from a simple description of the form of synaptic terminals and the molecules released from them to a more realistic discussion of the geometry of distribution of excitatory and inhibitory terminals on the surface of a neuron (Fig. 4.7a).

4.9 The geometry of synaptic endings

One approach to the geometry of synaptic endings can be made simply. When compared with a system for propagation of action potentials (over an axon for example) a synapse introduces into a

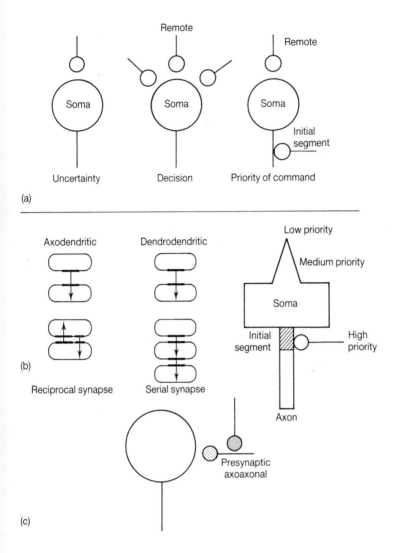

Fig. 4.7 (a) The geometry of synapses can be described simply in terms of the degree of uncertainty provided by the synapse, or more exactly the number of synapses needed to be involved in transmission. An element of decision making at synapses is shown by the need for summation of the effects generated by separate synaptic endings. Synapses on or close to the initial segment of the axon of a neuron have a greater priority of involvement in the decision-making process than those situated more remotely. (b) More exactly, the true geometry of synapses requires an added description of the structures involved in the synaptic array. The names are self-explanatory. An axon-making synapse with a dendrite of a neuron is described as axodendritic. (c) The presynaptic axoaxonal synapse (stippled) is able to modulate the amount of excitatory transmitter released by the synaptic terminals applied to the soma (the hatched ending). It is through this synaptic organization that presynaptic inhibition is mediated.

reflex system an important element of uncertainty (Fig. 4.7a). Not only has a stimulus to exceed the threshold of sensory receptors to initiate a motor response, it must generate an appropriate pattern of activity in the primary afferent axons of the sensory system and develop suitable postsynaptic potentials in the neuron somas involved.

The interaction of excitatory and inhibitory postsynaptic potentials (EPSPs and IPSPs) is an element of decision making in a nervous system (Fig. 4.7a). The position of any terminal on the soma of a neuron, for example, remote contact on a distant dendritic site or a contact with the initial segment on the axon (the site of initiation of an action potential) has a high priority for involve-ment in the decision-making processes in neural control.

4.10 From simple synaptic structure to circuits involving synapses

The oversimplified description of synaptic location on a 'billiard-ball' neuron soma (Fig. 4.7a) requires qualification. A synapse defined in terms of those neuronal structures making contact with each other leads us to a discussion of neuronal circuits and allows us to discuss the establishment of 'sets' of neurons through plastic adaptation.

When an axon terminal makes synaptic contact

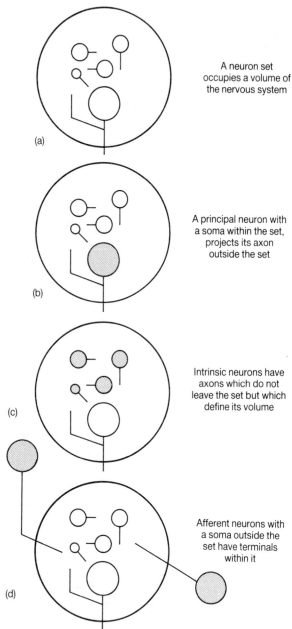

A neuron set occupies a volume of the nervous system

A principal neuron with a soma within the set, projects its axon outside the set

Intrinsic neurons have axons which do not leave the set but which define its volume

Afferent neurons with a soma outside the set have terminals within it

Fig. 4.8   A neuron set is a concept of the organization of neurons. Sets can be established during coherent neuronal activity by synaptic strengthening. It can occupy any volume of nervous system (a). The first definition of a set is based on the principal neurons it contains. These are the only neurons in the set whose axons leave its boundary (b). Intrinsic, or interneurons, are all contained within the set, and have axons that do not leave its boundary but determine its volume (c). Afferent neurons have axons which enter the set. These can come from structures central or peripheral to the set (d).

with a dendrite (Fig. 4.7b) an axodendritic contact is established. The names of synapse types 'axoaxonic and dendrodendritic' become clear from this example of definition. Reciprocal and axoaxo-dendritic synapses introduce the opportunity for neuron circuit formation and also indicate that interaction of synapses is feasible.

The arrows in Fig. 4.7b indicate the direction of transmission across the synapse. The terms pre-synaptic and postsynaptic apply as they did in Section 4.3.

It becomes apparent already in this section that the adaptive possibilities in the nervous system become great when the plasticity of synaptic action is admitted to the discussion. To understand fully the process of adaptive plasticity (adaptation refers here to the response of the neuromuscular system to a significant change in its environment or state compared with the definition in Section 4.5) we must introduce the concept of circuit formation using the example of neuron sets. The term was introduced in Section 4.5.

The sometimes confusing classical names of neurons, for example, Betz or Purkinje, and the perplexing variations in form neurons possess can be eliminated by identifying a role in neuron circuitry. A beginning of a discussion of circuitry starts with a definition of a set of neurons which occupies a volume of the nervous system. A principal neuron of the set projects an axon out of the set (cf. Fig. 4.8). One set can influence another set by means of this projection.

Intrinsic neurons have axons which remain within the volume of the set and incidentally define that volume. Input neurons transmit into the set from neural structures outside of it. These structures can be identified as sets of different composition.

> Big fleas have little fleas upon their backs to bite 'em and little fleas have lesser fleas and so *ad infinitum*.

Sets which develop through regular and consistent usage by motor controls, strengthen the interconnecting elements of the sets and become an important *unitary* component in the CNS.

4.11   Presynaptic inhibition

Strictly speaking, a discussion of presynaptic inhibition should not be included in a chapter describing synaptic transmission, but by doing so it introduces an understanding of the degree to which synaptic activity is controllable. An axoaxonic synapse (see Fig. 4.3 above) allows a modification of the release of the amount of an excitatory transmitter into the synaptic cleft. The release and therefore the effectiveness of the excitatory neurotransmitter of an afferent system can be decreased in this way or, more precisely, its contribution to the total excitatory effect on the target neuron can be decreased. This decrease leaves unchanged the excitatory/inhibitory interaction developed by postsynaptic influences. This topic will be discussed in relation to the development of the spastic states in Chapter 9.

References

Brown, M. L. and Hardman, W. J. (1987) Plasticity of vertebrate motoneurons. In: Winlow, W. and McCrohan, C. R. eds. *Growth and Plasticity of Neural Connections*. Manchester: Manchester University Press, pp. 35–55.

Bloom, W. and Fawcett, D. W. (1975) *A Textbook of Histology*. Philadelphia: W. B. Saunders.

Gutmann, E. (1969) The trophic functions of the nerve cell. *Scientia* **194**: 1–20.

Morrison, A. R. and Strick, P. L. (1983) *Changing Concepts of the Nervous System*. London: Academic Press.

Ochs, S. (1974) Systems of axoplasmic transport in nerve fibers (axonal transport) related to nerve function and trophic control. *Annals of the New York Academy of Sciences* **228**: 202–32.

Sherrington, C. S. (1906) *The Integrative Action of the Nervous System*. New Haven: Yale University Press.

Sherrington, C. S. (1913) Reflex inhibition in the control of movements and posture. *Quarterly Journal of Experimental Physiology* **6**: 255–310.

Tuffery, A. R. (1971) Growth and degeneration of motor endplates in normal cat limb muscles. *Journal of Anatomy* **110**: 221–47.

Vrbová, G, Gordon, T. and Jones, R. (1978) *Nerve–Muscle Interaction*. London: Chapman and Hall.

Vrbová, G. (1989) The concept of neuromuscular plasticity. In: Rose, F. C., Jones, R. and Vrbová, G. eds. *Comprehensive Neurologic Rehabilitation*. Volume 3: *Neuromuscular Stimulation: Basic Concepts and Clinical Implications*. New York: Demos.

Winlow, W. and McCrohan, C. R. (1987) *Growth and Plasticity of Neural Connections*. Manchester: Manchester University Press.

Chapter 5

Plasticity in development and redevelopment

5.1 Introduction

There are some 10 billion nerve cells in the brain, each of which makes 10 000 to a 100 000 contacts with other nerve cells – 1000 trillion connections in all. Yet despite these unimaginably large numbers, these connections are highly organized. Every centimetre of skin, for example, is innervated by nerve fibres that project to precise areas in somatosensory cortex in such an ordered way that a map of the body can be drawn on the cortex. There is also a large number of different types of neuron in the brain, each of which can be found in particular locations. Each cell has a characteristic pattern of dendritic and axonal arborization; each synthesizes and responds to characteristic neurotransmitters; each makes predictable connections with other cells. How do the cells find out what to become, which dendritic trees to grow, which transmitters to synthesize, and which connections to make?

The entire human genome probably contains about 100 000 genes, which is obviously insufficient to code specifically for the branching patterns and connections of each set of cells. It follows that the genes cannot contain a blueprint for the brain. Instead, the genes contain general instructions for growth guided by cues from the cell's environment. These local environmental cues turn relevant genes either on or off, and the processes coded for by the activated genes then interact with the environment to produce the differentiated cell.

It is important to realize that every cell in the body has all the genes coding for every other cell contained within its own nucleus. Obviously, most of these genes are switched off or toes would grow on the end of the nose, and worse. During devel-

opment, other specific parts of the genome are switched on to determine cell type and generate all of the characteristics of that type. In a consideration of plasticity one issue at stake is whether this is a once-and-for-all phenomenon or something that can be reactivated or changed with changing circumstances. A second issue is whether the processes encoded in the genes always produce the same result, or will different circumstances produce different results?

In this chapter, evidence will be presented that cells find out what to become and what connections to make on the basis of cues provided by their local environment. The opposite view is that cells become what their ancestry tells them to become. Evidence will also be presented to support the view that the branching pattern of neurites, the cells with which they connect and the effectiveness of these connections all change with use or after injury. The opposite view is that the strength and specificity of connections is laid down during embryological development and that thereafter there is only loss and degeneration.

5.2 The cerebral cortex and its development

5.2.1 Normal cortical histology

This section is a very brief outline of connections of the cerebral cortex, so that its plasticity can be discussed. Skilled histologists can persuade themselves that the neurons of the cortex are arranged in six layers. The outer or more superficial three layers evolved after the inner, deeper three layers, and they have different connections. The superficial layers of cells connect one part of the cortex to another, either in the same cerebral hemisphere (in which case they are called association fibres), or in the opposite hemisphere (in which case they are called commissural fibres). By contrast, the deeper neurons, which evolved much earlier, connect the cortex to subcortical structures and their axons are called projection fibres.

5.2.2   Normal cortical development

Cortical cells are born in the deepest layer of the developing forebrain, called the subventricular zone. They have to migrate through a layer of white matter and then enter the cortex proper, which is called the cortical plate at this stage. The first question to ask is 'How do the neurons know whether to become superficial cells with intracortical connections, or deep cells with subcortical connections?'

Fortunately for the neurons, the task of finding their way from the subventricular zone to the cortical plate is simplified by the presence of glial cells with long processes extending all the way from the subventricular zone, through the cortical plate, to the superficial covering of the brain known as the pia mater. These cells are called radial glia. Migrating neurons simply attach themselves to the radial glia, travel along their processes until they reach the cerebral cortex, and then detach themselves when they reach the appropriate cortical layer.

Now for a technical detour. When a cell divides it has to synthesize twice as much DNA as it had before, half for each daughter cell. This is the only time that large quantities of DNA are synthesized. The building blocks of DNA can be made radioactive, and a pulse of such radioactive building blocks can be given to an animal. We can be reasonably confident that any cells that take up much radioactivity have been dividing in the presence of the pulse. In this way, cells that divide at a specified time can be labelled. In other words, we can mark cells according to their birthdays.

Back to cortical development. Using this radioactive technique, it has been shown that cells which divide early on in foetal life migrate only to the deepest layers of the cortex and ultimately form subcortical connections. Cells which divide near the end of gestation, on the other hand, migrate as far as the superficial cortical layers where they form

cortico–cortical connections. Thus the capacity of the cortex to communicate with the rest of the brain evolved early and develops early, in deeper layers, whereas the capacity for intracortical communications, representing the degree of cortical processing, evolved later on and develops last, in the superficial layers. It would be interesting to know if early developmental defects affecting projection neurons result in different disorders from later developmental defects affecting association neurons. Could this be part of the difference between mental handicap without motor impairment, on the one hand, and motor disability without loss of intelligence on the other? But this is speculation.

5.2.3   Specification of cell type

There are clues about how cells know what to become. One clue is provided by mice called 'reeler' mice. They suffer from a hereditary disorder which makes them stagger. The basic defect is that while the cortical neurons born early on are well able to attach themselves to radial glia, they are unable to detach themselves again. As a result, they continue migrating along the radial glia until they reach the end of the glial processes, which brings them to the superficial layers of cortex. Consequently, the cortical neurons born later in development are unable to migrate to the superficial layers because the available space is already occupied by earlier neurons. The later neurons are forced to leave the radial glia in deeper layers of cortex than usual.

What will these neurons do? Will the early neurons take on the cortico–cortical connections of superficial neurons or will they remember that they should have been deep cells and project to subcortical targets? Will the later neurons, forced into a deep location, acquire the subcortical projections characteristic of deep neurons, or will they retain the cortico–cortical connections that their birth dates predict?

The answer is that the early neurons retain subcortical projections and the connections of late neurons are cortico–cortical. Clearly the final location of the neurons changes nothing and the birthday of the neuron is all that is required to predict the connections. Does this mean that connections are predetermined and that the cellular environment has no effect? Another set of experiments suggests that this is not the case. What may be important is the environment where the cell is born, not the environment where it finally settles.

The experiments which suggest that this might be the case involve transplantation of neurons from one animal at an early stage of development into the brain of another animal which has reached a much later stage of development. The transplanted neurons, born during the donor's early development, should migrate to deep levels of the host's cortex if their own birth date is the sole determining factor. On the other hand, the host cortex is at a late stage of development, so if environment is the sole determining factor the transplanted cells should migrate to superficial locations in the way that late cells normally do.

Before being removed from the host, the cells to be transplanted are labelled with a pulse of radioactive thymidine, one of the building blocks of DNA. When the host cortex is examined after transplantation of donor cells, the initially puzzling result is that some of the radioactive transplants have migrated to superficial locations whereas others are more deeply placed. Significantly, very few are found halfway between the deep and superficial locations. It is unlikely that half the transplanted cells are behaving in a predertermined way while the other half are environmentally determined, so what is the explanation? The answer is not yet certain, but a possible explanation involves the time it takes for a cell to complete its final cell division. This is of the order of 24 hours. The cells were removed from the host four hours after being pulse labelled. Thus some of them will have been in the final stages of cell division when they were removed, but others will only just have begun the process, which they will complete in the host brain. It follows that the former will finish dividing in an environment containing cues for early, deep cells, while the latter will complete their last division in an environment signalling that they are late, superficial cells. None will finish dividing in an environment telling them that they are of an intermediate age, destined for an intermediate depth. The subventricular zone environment may therefore be the critical cue to cell destiny: cells born in an early environment will become deep cells whereas cells born in a late environment will become superficial cells.

It appears, then, that whatever their type, the neurons in a vertical column of the cortex are all daughters of a single grandmother cell in the subventricular zone. They acquire differences from each other because the state of the subventricular zone changes with time, and the state prevailing on their birthday will determine what kind of cell each neuron will become. This stands in contrast to the alternative expectation that each kind of cell is the daughter of a different grandmother cell, specific to that cell type. Thus even in the very nature of individual cells, plasticity is at work, driving an early cell along one developmental path and a later cell along a different path, although they are both offspring of a single parent.

5.2.4 Developmental specification of connections

It has been seen above that the neurons from deep cortical layers project to subcortical targets. Not all the neurons in deep layers project to the same target, however. For example, neurons in motorsensory cortex project to the spinal cord whereas neurons in the visual cortex project to the dorsal part of the midbrain, called the superior colliculus or tectum. How do the cells know where to send their axons? Do they send fibres out at random, with those that happen to hit the target surviving, while other less accurate cells die? Or are they guided to the right target and nowhere else? Or do most cells send branches to most targets, later losing the inappropriate connections?

To answer this question, it is necessary to take another technological detour. Modern tract tracing techniques make the neurons do the work. A tracer, such as a fluorescent dye, is placed in one part of the brain. Fibres entering that part of the brain will take up the dye and transport it backwards towards the cell body, so that the body will be full of fluorescent tracer and can therefore be found. There is a blue tracer which labels the cytoplasm and a yellow tracer which labels the nucleus.

If this experiment is done on an adult with, say, a blue tracer injected into the spinal cord and a yellow tracer injected into the tectum, then the cytoplasm of neurons in the motorsensory cortex will become blue after transport of the dye backwards along their axons, whereas the nucleus of neurons in the visual cortex will take on a yellow colour. This is how it is known what the connections of these two areas are. If, on the other hand, the experiment is done on animals early in development, the rather startling result is that both sets of neurons have both dyes in them. The conclusion is that both motorsensory and visual cortex project initially to both tectum and spinal cord. Later in development the inappropriate connections are lost, leaving the adult pattern. Individual neurons therefore hedge their bets by projecting to widely different areas and only later shed unwanted collaterals, leaving connections with the adult pattern intact.

But where does the signal for pruning inappropriate connections come from? Does the cortex itself contain the information, or is it derived from elsewhere? To find this out, another transplantation experiment is required. A block of visual cortex from a young embryo is transplanted to the motorsensory area of another animal. Will the transplanted block of tissue contain within itself the information determining a tectal connection, typical of visual cortex? Or will the motorsensory cortical environment into which the block is placed dictate the retention of the spinal connection and deletion of the tectal connection? In short, is the final connection predetermined by a cell's ancestry or acquired from its environment?

When this experiment is done it turns out that, despite its visual origins, the transplanted block of cortex acquires projections to the spinal cord and loses those to the tectum. The connections are not predetermined from within the cortical block but related to the environment in which the block is placed. What, then, tells a block of cortical tissue where it is?

Apart from a small number of fibres originating in the brain stem, most axons that reach the cerebral cortex have come from the thalamus, which acts as the gateway to the cortex. The thalamus has many nuclei, each with a different input and each with a specific cortical destination. For example, one nucleus, ventralis posterior, has a somatic sensory input from the spinal cord and projects to the postcentral gyrus or somatosensory cortex. Another, the lateral geniculate nucleus, receives its input from the retina and projects to striate or visual cortex. A third receives its input from the inferior colliculus, a nucleus in the auditory pathway, and it projects to the transverse temporal gyri or auditory cortex.

This normal arrangement can be manipulated experimentally. The visual cortex is destroyed and the lateral geniculate nucleus dies by retrograde degeneration. The superior colliculus is also destroyed, so that the intact retina is deprived of both its normal targets. At the same time, the spinal projections to the ventroposterior thalamic

nucleus are destroyed, leaving the intact thalamocortical link to somatosensory cortex with no input. The embryo now has two problems: an intact visual input but no visual target and an intact somatosensory cortex but no somatosensory input. The two problems can be solved by a single stroke. The retinal cells with no target find the ventroposterior cells with no input and a complete, but abnormal, pathway from peripheral receptor to sensory cortex is established. The extraordinary thing is that the neurons in the somatosensory cortex now behave as if they were in the visual cortex, responding to light and generating visually evoked behaviour.

A similar experiment on ferrets involves removing the visual cortex and superior colliculus, as before, but this time destroying the inferior colliculus. In this case it is the medial geniculate nucleus and the auditory cortex that are intact but have no input. Once again the problem is solved by the retinal cells without a target finding the medial geniculate nucleus without an input. The auditory cortex takes on the properties of visual cortex and the ferret apparently 'sees' with its 'auditory' cortex. Of course, we cannot find out if the ferret 'hears' the light or 'sees' it. Operationally, however, it appears to be seeing.

In how many people with developmental brain disease has something like this actually happened? Perhaps positron emission tomographic (PET) scans will provide an answer. If the visual pathway has found its way to auditory cortex, then further damage of the 'auditory' cortex would lead to visual rather than auditory impairment. In other words if the plasticity of development shown to occur experimentally in other mammals also occurs in humans, it would make diagnosis of additional lesions somewhat unpredictable. None of the normal brain maps could be relied upon to predict lesion site in people with developmental aberrations. Consequently, each case would have to be treated as unique.

From the scientific point of view, however, these experiments indicate how the remarkable congruence of receptor mapping to sensory cortex might have been achieved. The cortex does not need to specify on a cell-to-cell basis where each part of a sensory path has to terminate. Instead, sensory information reaching the cortex via the thalamus is, in itself, sufficient to determine how the receiving cortical cells will react. The pathways responding to stimulation of the thumb, for instance, determine that the cortical cells at their point of arrival will represent the thumb. This is more plausible than assuming that some cortical cells are predestined to respond to the thumb, in which case afferents from the thumb would have to find them. Such a hypothesis requires that literally millions of cells would each have a different label which could be detected and differentiated by the incoming fibres, an unimaginably difficult task.

The changes we have just looked at are gross changes involving substitution of one afferent modality for another. The interaction of adjacent fibres belonging to the same modality also needs to be considered. What happens if two fibres arrive in the same part of the cortex?

Two important principles in development and redevelopment are concerned with, first, competition between rival groups of fibres, and, second, synergism within one group. Initially, when two pathways converge on the same target, their fibres are intermingled, so that no part of the innervated territory is obviously the exclusive province of either set of inputs. It can be expected that fibres in one pathway will fire more synchronously with each other than with the fibres of the other pathway, simply because they will be exposed to more similar stimulation. Considering any particular zone of the innervated territory, the chances are that, from time to time, nearly synchronous activity will occur within neighbouring fibres of one pathway but not the other. At a critical stage in development this will lead to mutual strengthening of the synchronous synapses in that zone, with a concomitant weakening of the synapses of the other pathway. As a result, the dominant group retains its stabilized synapses whereas the less synchronous group loses its projection to the zone. Meanwhile, the reverse will occur in other zones of the innervated territory, the second pathway capturing the zone to the detriment of the first pathway. It is like a playground filled with two rival gangs. Initially, the members of each gang are dispersed all over the playground, struggling to gain the upper hand. Gradually, however, pockets will emerge where in some cases one gang has the advantage, in other cases the converse. Territory is gained and held. By mutual support between fibres of the same pathway and competition against the fibres of the opposing pathway, the innervated territory is eventually divided into interlocking zones, each zone being dominated by one or other pathway.

As always, there is nothing predestined in this partition. Any overall reduction in the activity of one of the pathways will lead to a corresponding restriction in the sizes of the zones it eventually captures. The rival pathway, with undiminished activity, will expand its territory to occupy the margins of the zones vacated by the weaker input. Thick stripes belonging to the active pathway will alternate with thin stripes innervated by the less active pathway. Once again, the brain adapts plastically to the actual circumstances confronting its own development, and there is no slavish following of a master blueprint rigidly laid down for all brains at all times regardless of their individual histories. The brain grows to suit its own reality.

It is evident, then, that the astonishing degree of organization in the cerebral cortex, with maps of the retina, cochlea, skin and joints precisely arranged along its surface, has not come about by reading an exact blueprint from the genes. It is now clear that the genes simply specify the rules governing how one cell interacts with another and with the matrix of extracellular molecules around it. By reading the cues so obtained, functional groupings, or sets of cells, literally make themselves. The amazing precision of the correspondence between peripheral receptor surfaces and their cortical representation is now seen to be the consequence of flexible development, with cells taking on the properties that local opportunities present. No rigid master plan is being imposed here, but each cell jostles with its neighbours until their collective interaction plastically creates the order essential to the whole. This individualistic anarchy may not work for people, but it seems to work for nerve cells.

5.2.5 Redevelopment of connections

The previous work indicates that brain maps of sensory surfaces arise initially from the pattern of information reaching the sensory cortex during the critical developmental period. If the pattern changes in adult life, will the brain map change too? The cortical representation of a monkey's hand has been used to answer this question. The skin of a monkey's hand is represented in an ordered pattern in the somatosensory cortex, with the representation of the thumb next to that of the index finger, then the middle finger and so on. If some heroic experimenter taps the monkey's index and middle fingers, but no others, for an hour or two a day for several months, changes in the cortical representation of the fingers are induced. The region of cortex devoted to processing tactile information from the tapped fingers increases, distorting the map in favour of these two digits. This happens in adult monkeys, and it is likely to happen to us. Using a part of the body more frequently causes it to be given greater cortical representation. This may be one of the ways in which constant practice improves performance; proprioceptors from muscles and joints subjected to increased stimulation might well acquire an enlarged area of cortical representation, leading to improved use of the parts in question.

The example just given involves stimulation of a relatively 'normal' or 'physiological' kind. Peripheral nerve injury provides another means of altering the input from the skin. The median nerve innervates the palmar surface of the first three and a half digits, but the radial nerve innervates the dorsal surface of the first two and a half. Obviously the palmar surface of the hand is more frequently stimulated than the dorsal surface, and correspondingly, the palmar surface of an intact monkey's hand has a larger area of cortical representation than the dorsal surface.

This can be changed by cutting the median nerve. Now the cortical cells have no tactile input from the median nerve, but instead of dying or doing nothing, they begin to respond to the input from the radial nerve. The cortical area representing the denervated palmar surface shrinks, giving ground to the representation of the dorsal surface. Clearly the cortex works on the principle 'if you don't use it, you lose it'.

If, now, the median nerve is sutured and allowed to reinnervate the palmar surface, it is able to recapture some of its lost territory. The radial nerve, though, is able to retain some of the territory it gained before reinnervation took place. Recovery is probably incomplete because reinnervation through a sutured nerve is never exact, axons finding their way down inappropriate channels or getting caught up in connective tissue scars. On the other hand, crushing the median nerve allows almost perfect reinnervation because each regenerated axon grows down exactly the right channel. In this case the median nerve succeeds in a nearly total recapture of its lost territory and the *status quo ante* is fully restored.

These changes outlined so far are macroscopic changes, seen in populations of cells, but similar plasticity can also be observed at the cellular level.

An example concerns the pattern of dendritic trees in the motorsensory cortex. Individual rats prefer to use one paw rather than the other. If a rat prefers to use, say, the right paw, then the cells of the motorsensory cortex of the left hemisphere will have rich, profusely branched dendritic trees. By contrast, cells in the motorsensory cortex on the right side, representing the less used left paw, will have shorter, less frequently branched dendritic trees. Although this might appear to be the anatomical basis of paw preference, caution is required: causation in the brain is inherently circular, as we shall see.

Laboratory rats are cooperative creatures and they can be persuaded to use a less preferred paw, let us say the left, in return for some reward. With training, the rat eventually switches to using the left paw. If the cortex of a rat is examined after such training, it will be found that the poor, stunted dendritic shrubs in the right motorsensory cortex have blossomed into profusely branching trees. Conversely, the formerly richly branched trees of the left side have now shrunk, losing both length and degree of branching. Once again, a 'use it or lose it' principle is at work.

What do these changes in dendritic trees imply? If the number of synapses per unit area of dendritic surface is constant, a larger dendritic tree will have more synapses on it. These may be more synapses with those axons which were previously connected to it, in which case it will respond more vigorously to the input it had before. Alternatively, the synapses may be with previously unconnected axons, in which case it will have a more varied input. The cell will therefore be better at what it previously did, and it will also do more. The repertoire of this cell will thereby become richer, and the role of the function it represents will be increased, all by plastic adaptation.

There are many examples of such changes, not just in the cortex, nor only in experimental animals. Purkinje cells from the cerebellum and striatal cells from the basal ganglia both show analagous changes. When the brains of active people are examined, these cell types show greater dendritic trees with more spines and longer segments than cells taken from inactive people. Cortical neurons from people who are assumed to have had a richer intellectual environment have greater dendritic trees than people with less intellectually demanding jobs. Of course, with human material, causation is always a problem: it can be argued that the people with more branched dendrites were thereby permitted to become more active, or that both activity and greater dendritic branching are the result of a third factor such as better nutritional status. Animal experiments, however, allow causation to be manipulated directly and these experiments generally show that while greater dendritic branching may well cause increased activity, the converse also holds: greater activity causes greater dendritic branching. Cause creates effect which alters the cause. To reiterate, causality in the brain is inherently circular.

In this section, evidence that the function of a part of the cortex, the patterns of branching of neurons and the connections they make can all be changed in the adult has all been presented. Such things are not laid down indelibly at the start of life, but continually alter in response to changes in use and experience.

5.3   Altering the strength of existing synapses

The previous section dealt with making new connections between neurons, but plasticity is not confined to anatomical changes. It can be shown that the effectiveness of a synapse which already exists can be changed too. One way in which this can happen is called post-tetanic potentiation. It is well established that action potentials are generally of a constant, unvarying size. Typically, action potentials are found in axons. Potentials in dendrites can sometimes have the unvarying characteristics of an action potential, but more usually they are graded. Dendritic potentials also propagate in a different way and they can be added to and subtracted from each other, allowing cellular computation to occur. From the perspective of plasticity, however, a very interesting property is that they can vary in amplitude in response to the same input.

If a presynaptic cell is weakly stimulated, the postsynaptic cell will respond with a postsynaptic potential of a given amplitude. If, after a delay, the presynaptic cell is again stimulated, the amplitude of the postsynaptic cell will be the same as before. Nothing plastic has happened and classical neuroscientists sleep comfortably in their beds. If, however, the presynaptic cell is stimulated to fire at a greater frequency, successive postsynaptic potentials will begin before the immediately preceding one has died down and they will therefore be superimposed on each other, adding in amplitude. This

is called temporal summation. If, after a delay of up to a few hours, a single presynaptic potential is evoked, the amplitude of the postsynaptic potential this time will be greater than before. This enhancement of the postsynaptic potential's amplitude is called posttetanic potentiation. As far as learning is concerned it is not the solution to the memory trace because it lasts only a few hours.

There is, however, a superficially similar phenomenon called long-term potentiation. Like post-tetanic potentiation, it is induced by high-frequency discharge of the presynaptic cell. The principal difference, though, is that long-term potentiation lasts for days, weeks and perhaps even months. It is a much more likely candidate for the biological basis of some kinds of learning.

What are the characteristics of long-term potentiation? To serve as a model of learning it has to have specificity: learning that a bell signals the arrival of food does not imply that any and all sounds signal food. In the same way, if one of two afferents to a cell is stimulated sufficiently to cause long-term potentiation, later testing of the other afferent does not evoke an enhanced postsynaptic response. Only the specific response to the stimulated input shows an increased amplitude.

Another feature of associative learning is that when two stimuli occur together in the correct temporal sequence, one stimulus acquires the capacity to stand for the other and elicit the same responses. Long-term potentiation also has this associative property. If neither of two afferents to a cell has an input powerful enough to induce long-term potentiation, stimulation of both afferents simultaneously may well achieve the desired effect; the two afferents have now become associated, one afferent becoming capable of evoking the postsynaptic amplitude to be expected from stimulating both together. In this case, spatial summation between two weak inputs has served the purpose of temporal summation in one strong input.

The importance of long-term potentiation is that it provides an example of how already existing synapses can change their effectiveness over durations long enough to be relevant to learning. A well-used route through the brain becomes more effective through long-term potentiation. Furthermore, an ineffective route converging on an effective route, can, if simultaneously active, acquire the capacity to substitute for the effective route. Finally, two ineffective routes can mutually potentiate each other, so that both can now evoke activity downstream from their point of convergence. In chapter 8, the mechanisms thought to underlie long-term potentiation will be elucidated, and it will become evident that some of these mechanisms are remarkably similar to those responsible for development. If so, learning can be thought of as redevelopment of the brain. The process of building connections and strengthening them is continuous, never ceasing from the moment the first synapse sputters into life until the final synaptic exchange takes place.

5.4 Plastic changes after injury

It was shown above that injury to the developing brain reveals a considerable capacity to reorganize the growth of connections while they are still being formed. It was also shown that 'physiological' changes in the use of an adult neuron can alter its morphology and the strength of its synapses. Perhaps of most interest to therapists, however, is the extent to which such changes can take place after injury in an already formed brain. Not many years ago, the conventional wisdom was that attempts to rearrange and regrow the adult nervous system were always abortive. In the last decade or so, by contrast, an overwhelming wealth of data has demolished the view that the adult nervous system is fixed and unchanging. This section outlines some of the concepts involved.

5.4.1 Changes brought about by damage to a cell's afferents

In tissue culture, neurons will express their usual morphology, indicating that the information for the pattern of dendritic and axonal branching is contained within the cell. Nevertheless, this does not mean that the pattern of branching is fixed and immutable. It has already been said that a normal reduction in the input to a neuron alters its morphology: not using a formerly preferred paw leads to atrophy of the corresponding dendritic tree in the motorsensory cortex of rats. Destruction of the afferents to a neuron is a more drastic reduction of input than disuse. As expected, the dendritic tree is altered. Minor loss of input leads to collapse of spines into the dendritic shafts which bear them but, provided other afferents remain intact, the dendrite itself survives. If, however, there is a more extensive destruction of a neuron's afferents, then dendrites also shrink. This shrinkage is specific to the dendritic region denervated: if one part of the dendritic tree is denervated, then only that part atrophies, leaving innervated parts of the tree intact. Whatever process is responsible for the shrinkage, it is exactly matched to the degree of deprivation, affecting only those precise parts of the arbour that no longer have significant input. It is not usual to consider such changes as being plastic, but they are changes in phenotype in response to altered local environment, and as such they can be seen as a form of plastic adaptation.

With severe loss of a large part of the neuron's afferents there is a more general effect. In this case, the denervated neuron undergoes total degeneration, no part of it surviving. Thus the morphology of a neuron is plastically matched to its input, to the extent that if there is little significant input the neuron dies. This process, whereby an uninjured cell dies in consequence of injury to its afferent neurons, is called transneuronal degeneration. A transneuronally degenerated cell will in its turn deprive its target neurons of part of their input. In widely ramifying circuits, characterized by a multiplicity of inputs from different sources, degeneration at one point in the circuit will lead to no more than atrophy of the secondarily denervated dendrites of the next cell in the chain. In closed systems, however, where a significant part of the input to the next cell in the chain comes from transneuronally degenerated cells, the next cell will itself degenerate. Transneuronal degeneration will therefore permeate through a closed circuit by knock-on effects, and successive neurons in the chain will die as they lose the input from preceding cells.

It is important to realize that the clinical manifestation of a lesion of the nervous system may not be a direct result of the injury, but represent transneuronal loss further down a chain of neurons. An obvious strategy for therapists is to know in detail what inputs to a set of partially denervated neurons survive, and to direct therapy towards optimally stimulating these remaining inputs, in the hope of minimizing secondary transneuronal degeneration. Of course, this requires, first, a precise knowledge of the site of the lesion; second, an extensive knowledge of the neuroanatomy and the functions of the circuits involved; and, third, techniques to increase activity in specific circuits. Finally, careful appraisal of the consequences of such strategies needs to be made. It may well be, for example, that increased activity in a damaged circuit will lead to greater damage, while reduced activity allows the metabolism to be directed towards repair processes. The optimal balance between these opposing factors has to be determined empirically. It will be different in different circuits and after different lesions, because it will depend on the ratio of remaining excitation and inhibition.

5.4.2 Changes brought about by damage to a cell's output

The least damaging change to a cell's output is destruction of the target before the axon has reached it. This leaves the cell in question uninjured. We have seen some of the consequences of experimental injury of this kind in the section on development: a sensory neuron deprived of its normal target can find new structures to innervate. A further example is the retinotectal pathway, involved in generating movements of the eyes and head in response to crudely processed visual stimuli. Normally the retina projects directly to the part of the midbrain called the superior colliculus. Removal of the superior colliculus on one side before the arrival of optic fibres results in the growing fibres rerouting themselves to the intact side. All is well, except that when the animal later responds to visual stimuli, it may misdirect the response to the wrong side.

The next degree of damage involves a lesion of axons. In the developing nervous system, such an injury can be surmounted by simply rerouting the growing fibres around the injury. Injury to the spinal cord, for example, interrupts the route for corticospinal fibres. The injured region can be bypassed so that the corticospinal axons reach their normal target by an abnormal route, and the experimental animal is apparently none the worse for the injury.

In adult mammals, however, the outcome is less sanguine. Regrowth of myelinated axons in the adult central nervous system (CNS) is extremely limited. The greatest distance over which regrowth succeeds is less than 100 μm, or a tenth of a millimetre. Possible reasons for this will be discussed in Chapter 8. What happens to a cell with a damaged axon? In fact, similar principles apply to axonal damage as have been described for damage to a cell's afferents. For an extensively arborizing axon, loss of a small part of the axonal tree has no great effect on the cell. Indeed, surviving axonal branches may increase the number of synapses they make elsewhere, much as a pruned bush will grow more densely below the cut.

If, on the other hand, the damaged part of the axon is a considerable portion of its total arborization, the situation is different. The cell appears to lack some vital signal from its target, and it closes down. Its genes are no longer transcribed into messenger RNA, so the Nissl substance of the cell disappears, translation of genetic information into protein synthesis stops and eventually the cell dies. This is retrograde degeneration. If the inputs to the retrogradely degenerated cell have other irons in the fire, sending branches elsewhere, that is the end of the matter. If, however, the degenerated cell was part of a closed circuit, so that its afferents have no other target neurons, then they too will suffer from deprivation of vital signal from their target and they will also die. Thus retrograde degeneration in a closed circuit can result in transneuronal degeneration of successively earlier cells in the pathway. Once again, clinical symptoms may be more the result of loss of these secondarily damaged cells than of the original lesion. An example of this is seen following damage to the limbic cortex (Bleier, 1969): loss of limbic cortex leads to degeneration of the anterior nucleus of the thalamus which leads in turn to loss of the mamillary bodies. This circuit is the one damaged in amnesic syndromes, for example, following chronic alcoholism or deficiency of thiamine, a vitamin.

5.4.3 Changes brought about by damage in neighbouring cells

The changes described above, although negative, can be seen as a plastic adaptation of the nervous system, remodelling cells to remove parts of a circuit that are no longer active. By themselves, they are no great cause for excitement. What has caught the collective imagination is the more positive aspects of plastic adaptation, where new growth occurs.

If part of the total input to a nucleus is lost, surviving fibres replace them. This has been termed reactive synaptogenesis in the case of surviving fibres that are neighbours of the lost input, and axonal sprouting when the fibres come from outside the immediate region of damage. The effect of this replacement depends on the nature of the circuit. In topographically precise circuits, where the position of a fibre in a tract is part of the information conveyed by that fibre, replaced synapses may blur the acuity of the system, perhaps increasing the handicap. On the other hand, in those circuits where topographical relations are uninformative, replacement of a lost fibre by its neighbours may successfully restore function. This is characteristic of those systems that act by diffusion of neurotransmitters over relatively long distances.

Lost afferents to a denervated territory may be replaced by fibres that come from outside the territory. This is sometimes distinguished from reactive synaptogenesis on the grounds that the new connections are different in kind. Obviously, if the new connections are with fibres that normally have a totally different kind of function, then the message they transmit into the damaged circuit may be gibberish and lead to a further impairment of function. Even when the information they bring is not totally different in kind, it may lead to an undesirable disharmony. For example, after transaction of the spinal cord, the number of synapses on neurons below the lesion is decreased, corresponding to loss of descending tracts. After an interval of weeks to months, however, the number of synapses on each cell gradually builds up until it may reach prelesion levels, at which point no further increase occurs. Where have the new synapses come from?

They can come from only two sources: either interneurons or primary afferents. Their consequence is that what was previously only part of the input to a cell, balanced by descending fibres, is now the total input with an increased strength. Activation of the relevant afferents now has a greater effect than before, simply because there are more synapses conveying the same information. It would be somewhat surprising if this compensatory increase in the synaptic strength of afferents and interneurons did not contribute at least in part to the hyperreflexia seen after cord transection (see chapter 6). Thus plasticity of the nervous system may not always be desirable. In fact, contrary to previous dogma, plasticity may be very widespread and contribute substantially to the total clinical deficit by generating spurious synapses conveying only disruptive disinformation or unbalancing normal information. The harm done will be particularly marked in circuits with precise topographical relationships. More beneficial effects might be expected in circuits that do not depend on precise anatomical relationships.

Examples of these latter systems are the noradrenergic, dopaminergic, serotonergic and cholinergic systems. These systems frequently lack conventional synapses and the transmitter is simply released into the extracellular fluid and diffuses to target neurons that are not in direct synaptic contact with the releasing terminal. Such systems are more like local 'hormonal' or endocrine systems than conventional neural circuits. Because the transmitter does not actually enter the blood stream, they are not truly hormonal or endocrine, so they are termed paracrine instead. Whereas spatially informative systems act rapidly and briefly through ligand gated voltage channels, paracrine systems frequently act through second messengers with delayed, prolonged affects.

It is no coincidence that these are predominantly the systems which have been amenable to drug therapy: drugs are usually delivered in such a way that they enter the brain without any sharp spatial localization, and it is mainly in these paracrine systems lacking strict spatial information that drugs can work successfully. For spatially dependent pathways, delivery of a drug to all parts of the system simultaneously would act as a biochemical sledgehammer, causing more disruption than restoration of function. It is also in these paracrine systems of the brain that transplantation is more likely to restore function, for the same reasons.

5.5 Grafting and transplantation

One of the arguments against plasticity in the adult brain was that mature neurons were thought to have lost the capacity to grow. This assertion was an early casualty of the renewed investigation of plasticity. It is by now well known that after transection of the spinal cord, a peripheral nerve can be grafted across the lesion and central neurons will grow into both ends of the graft for distances of up to 3 cm. More recently, similar experiments have shown that retinal neurons will grown down a peripheral nerve graft all the way to the superior colliculus, which they enter and successfully innervate, even in an adult animal. Lack of long distance growth is therefore certainly not the result of an absolute inability of mature central neurons to grow. The answer lies in the effect of mature neuropil on mature neurons, as will be discussed in more detail in chapter 8.

The idea that immature neuropil may be more conducive to the growth of adult axons has led to a number of experiments in which blocks of immature nervous tissue are transplanted into a lesioned pathway in a mature brain. The disrupted pathway can regenerate through the immature graft and the mature cells are partly sustained by contact with it. After spinal cord transection, for example, rubrospinal neurons normally degenerate. If a foetal transplant is inserted into the lesion, rubrospinal fibres grow into it and some of the rubrospinal neurons are thereby able to survive. Similarly, descending serotonergic fibres are also able to cross a foetal graft and survive (Bregman, 1987).

Transplants not only serve to sustain surviving fibres of a lesioned host, but they can also replace lost neurons altogether. This is especially obvious in paracrine neural systems. It is now well publicized that transplantation of foetal substantia nigra into adults with damaged nigrostriatal tracts can restore function following the growth of connections with the host striatum. This has been shown experimentally in rats and monkeys, but despite some early successes, the results in humans are less clear cut. No doubt the preconditions for success need to be more thoroughly studied and the cell biology of the processes involved understood in greater depth before this becomes a routine therapy, assuming other technologies do not supercede it first.

5.6 Conclusion

This chapter has attempted to provide an overview of the phenomena of plasticity in the CNS. Although purists, bound to exact definitions, may disagree, an attempt has been made to blur the distinctions between initial growth of the nervous system, change with experience and regrowth after injury. These three processes may not be exactly the same, occurring as they do in different contexts and induced by different pressures, but there is an underlying similarity in the cellular and molecular events that bring them about, as chapter 8 will endeavour to demonstrate. The principal message of this chapter is that the brain does not grow once and for all during development, then show no further change except degeneration in adult life. It is undergoing a continuous remodelling at both molecular and cellular levels. Its connections, transmitter levels, receptors, dendritic and axonal arborizations are all in a dynamic state of flux, being built up and torn down in a precise, controlled response to changes in the use and experience of the brain. It is, in fact, living tissue. Minds may lack plasticity, but brains do not.

References

Agnati, L. F., Zini, I., Zoli, M., Fuxe, K., Merlo Pich, E., Grimaldi, R., Toffano, G. and Goldstein, M. (1988) Regeneration in the central nervous system: concepts and facts. *Advances in Tech Stand Neurosurgery* **16**: 3–50.

Bleier, R. (1969) Retrograde transsynaptic cellular degeneration in mamillary ventral tegmnental nuclei following limbic decortication in rabbits of various ages. *Brain Res.* **15**: 365–93.

Bregman, B. S. (1987) Spinal cord transplants permit the growth of serotonergic axons across the site of neonatal spinal cord transection. *Brain Res.* **431**: 265–79.

Kaplan, M. S. (1988) Plasticity after brain lesions: contemporary concepts. *Archives of Physical Rehabilitation* **69**: 984–91.

Steward, O. (1989) Reorganization of neuronal connections following CNS trauma: principles and experimental design. *Journal of Neurotrauma* **6**: 99–152.

Chapter 6

A review of the neural control of movement

6.1 Introduction

Until now this book has presented a new physiology; one which involves more than just a stimulus–response outlook. However, this chapter will now look at the control of movement by the central nervous system (CNS) in terms of 'classical' stimulus–response physiology. The question may be asked: why do we need to look at 'classical' neurophysiology in an exposition on the plasticity of the neuromuscular system?

It has been suggested that 'to live is to change . . . ' and the neuromuscular system develops and changes due to the activity of the individual and in order to adapt to the environment. Once it has reached maturity it does not become static but continues to change in response to the environment and its own induced activity, particularly after damage. How the environment shapes the neuromuscular system initially and what it is when shaped is important if we are to understand how we can help to influence the shaping. How the environment continues to shape the system during maturity, through the effects of afferent input to the CNS is also important as these forces come into their own following damage to the CNS. These forces can be guided and assisted.

Current knowledge of stimulus–response physiology helps to explain how the CNS controls movement in the short term and how environmental influences help to determine responses. This knowledge should help us to determine the long-term effects of CNS activity in shaping the neuromuscular system. In the natural environment stimulus response is accompanied by a trophic effect which

changes or reinforces for the future. Artificially induced stimulus response may not contain this trophic code. The code must be identified if artificial stimulation is to be used. However, naturally occurring stimuli can be manipulated in order to achieve and reinforce the stimulus response but also the trophic effect. Stimulus response must first be described as it is known in relation to movement control before it can be manipulated to the benefit of the brain-damaged patient.

Therefore this chapter will discuss the phylogenetic and ontogenetic development of the nervous system control of movement. It will look at the role of the spinal cord in movement control and the effects of descending input from the brain and afferent input from the periphery on the spinal cord. A study of the role of afferent input from the periphery on the CNS control of movement is of particular importance if we are to understand how afferent input can be manipulated in order to guide the nervous system in its adaptation to a changing environment.

This chapter is an overview only and will look briefly at the role of higher centres within the brain in movement control. However, adequate references will be given for further study.

6.2 Scheme of movement control by the central nervous system

The control of movement by the CNS has been described as hierarchical (Jackson, 1884). Hughlings-Jackson described movements in terms of their degree of voluntary control, movements ranging from the most automatic to the least automatic. Although this may be an oversimplification, it still holds true that movements may be more or less automatic and that spinal movement is the most automatic. This scale from the most automatic to the least automatic is also seen in the development of the CNS, both phylogenetically and ontogenetically. For example, in ontogenetic development, the automatic postural adjustments controlled by the brain stem appear first in human infants, before the ability to execute the pinch–grip which requires a high degree of voluntary control as well as automatic postural adjustments.

The spinal cord as the region which produces the most automatic movement is capable, nevertheless, of producing all basic patterns of movement autonomously. The spinal cord also contains the circuitry necessary for all the more sophisticated movements and postural adjustments. The spinal cord has been described as the region for the execution of movement (see Fig. 6.1). The motor activities of the motorsensory cortex (Ms) direct the spinal cord to produce all these more sophisticated movements through its output to the muscles. The Ms therefore initiates and also modifies the output from the spinal cord. The Ms is able to work at the direction of other more highly developed regions of the brain and also through the direction of input from the periphery. Regions of the brain such as the basal ganglia and the premotor cortex store programmes of learned movements and can direct the Ms in the initiation of these learned programmes. These programming regions are also thought to direct automatic postural adjustments which accompany all voluntary movements and in some cases they do this by affecting the spinal cord through pathways other than direct cortico–spinal pathways. The Ms on receiving instructions from other higher brain centres decodes the programme information and informs the spinal cord of the action needed. Because of learned programmes complex movements can be carried out more efficiently.

Although the programming areas and the Ms can begin their chain of command through the development of an idea of movement in the frontal cortex, the chain can also be initiated through sensory input to other areas of the cerebral cortex. In normal movement the accompanying sensory input to the sensorymotor cortex (Sm) helps to direct and facilitate the movement but control is imposed by the other higher centres. The movement once begun is also accompanied by feedback to other

levels, for example, the spinal cord or cerebellum. This feedback can help in the adjustment of movement already in progress but it is important to appreciate that feedback to the spinal cord can initiate movement at spinal cord level, bypassing the Ms.

The brain stem is considered to be at an intermediate level in the hierarchy of movement control, one level above the spinal cord but below the motorsensory cortex and other higher centres (see Fig. 6.1). This is because many brain stem mechanisms are reflex actions of a slightly more sophisticated nature than spinal reflexes, often arising from special sensory receptors such as those in the labyrinths of the inner ear. Like the Ms the brain stem can affect the spinal cord to produce movement or changes in muscle tone but of an automatic nature rather than voluntary. Brain stem control could therefore be considered to act in parallel with cortical control as well as being at a lower level in the hierarchy. Ghez (1985) suggests that this parallel yet hierarchical organization is shown by the fact that the brain stem and motorsensory cortex can both directly affect the spinal cord and its execution of movement but the Ms can also control brain stem activity through its cortico–bulbar connections.

Support for a hierarchical control has developed through many studies carried out since it was first suggested by Hughlings-Jackson in 1884. However, it is still not possible to state categorically the role of different regions of the brain and their place in the hierarchy. Many ideas on the role of different regions have developed through lesion studies in humans. However, the loss of a particular function following a lesion to a part of the CNS does not mean that that region was responsible for the function. One explanation may be that the region may have acted as a link in the chain of command from the region actually responsible. Another explanation may be that the function is one of many carried out by the damaged part but it is the only one that cannot be taken over by other parts. This second explanation opens the door for the many theories of the recovery potential of the CNS and gives hope for the brain-injured patient.

6.3 Development of the nervous system control of movement

A study of the phylogeny of locomotion supports the idea of hierarchies of movement control. The

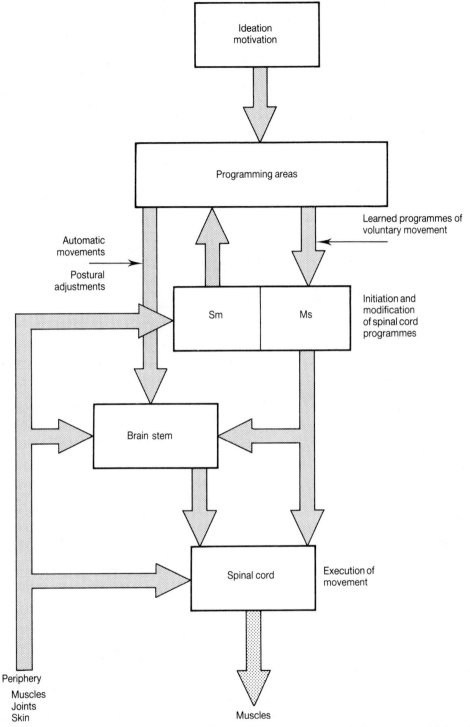

Fig. 6.1 The control of movement by the CNS shows a hierarchical yet parallel organization. (a) Spinal cord, brain stem, motorsensory cortex (Ms) and programming areas are at successively higher levels in the hierarchy. The spinal cord produces automatic reflex activity and basic programmes of movement; the brain stem produces more complex automatic reflex activity; the motorsensory cortex initiates and modifies spinal cord activity to produce voluntary movement; programming areas direct the Ms and the brain stem to influence the spinal cord. (b) The Ms acts on the spinal cord to produce voluntary movement; the brain stem acts on the spinal cord to produce automatic movements and postural adjustments which accompany voluntary movement; the input from the periphery acts on the spinal cord in conjuction with the Ms and the brain stem to support these regions in their activity. Sm: Sensorimotor cortex.

ability to move from place to place increased with the development of a skeleton and the ability to generate muscular force. The fish is able to swim through the alternate contraction of lateral flexor muscles and this is thought to occur through the activity of a movement or swimming generator within the nervous system. This would appear to be analogous to the movement generator hypothesized in the spinal cord of vertebrates which is capable of producing all basic locomotory patterns autonomously. Once the jointed skeleton and appendages had developed independently in arthropods and vertebrates then a greater ability to move by walking and to modify basic activity existed. The cockroach, an arthropod, was studied by Pearson in the 1970s and he was able to demonstrate the production of alternating flexor and extensor activity by the neuraxis similar to that occurring in the cat. This activity in the cockroach was considered to be under tonic excitatory drive by higher centres but was also shown to be capable of modification by afferent input (Pearson and Duysens, 1976). In the cat, many studies have demonstrated the ability of the spinal cord to produce basic locomotory patterns (see Grillner, 1981). These patterns have also been shown to be capable of modification by afferent input from the periphery and also by centres in the brain.

The development of brain stem mechanisms concerned with balance can be seen in the development of the otolith organs in the inner ear in vertebrates. This shows the development of a lower brain stem which can influence the movement generator in the spinal cord to modify output.

The development of the arm and hand in primates from the forelimbs of lower vertebrates shows how animals in their phylogeny have adapted to new environments or needs. The development of higher levels of CNS control commensurate with the needs of manipulation and the upright posture is also seen, and areas of the cerebellum and cerebral cortex are most highly developed in humans.

Ontogenetic development in humans sometimes reflects phylogenetic development. At birth the baby shows automatic walking, a reflex activity that occurs if the baby is held under the arms with the feet placed on a firm surface. This may persist for up to six weeks (Illingworth, 1987) and may be an indication of a spinal movement generator operating without any inhibition from higher centres. Many other examples of spinal reflex activity normally inhibited in the adult are seen in the new-

born, including the grasp response. This response is only seen in adults following damage to descending tracts resulting in spasticity. Righting reactions due to neck and labyrinthine brain stem reflexes begin to develop from birth and equilibrium reactions appear around the sixth month and gradually develop in different positions. More sophisticated postural adjustments which accompany voluntary movement and reflect control by centres higher than the brain stem appear much later. The pinch-grip attributed to an intact cortico-spinal tract usually develops by approximately 40 weeks after birth and has to be accompanied by automatic postural adjustments but these adjustments are not refined till much later. Equally, reaching movements will be inaccurate and ataxic for some time and the eye-hand coordination needed to catch a ball will take several years to develop. These sophisticated activities are examples of the high degree of movement control imposed by the higher levels of the hierarchy in primates, particularly in humans.

A study of phylogenetic and ontogenetic development aids in the understanding of the way in which the CNS controls movement but the knowledge is also helpful in the rehabilitation of brain-damaged children and adults. Perinatal damage to the CNS can cause an arresting or retardation of development so that ontogenetic development does not keep pace with chronological development. It can also lead to abnormal development which could be due either to a lack of peripheral influence on the CNS during development or to an abnormal influence. Because peripheral input due to movement helps to guide ontogenetic development it is essential that the child is encouraged to move in as normal a way as possible. It is also important to appreciate in the child and the adult with brain damage that aspects of motor control cannot exist in isolation; for example, the use of the hand for grasping or for more sophisticated manipulative procedures is impossible without the ability to initiate postural adjustments which must accompany the activity. The rest of this chapter will consider different levels of the hierarchy of movement control with particular emphasis on the effect of input from the periphery to the different levels.

6.4 Role of the spinal cord in movement

Early neurophysiological studies on spinal and decerebrate cats (Sherrington, 1910; Brown, 1911)

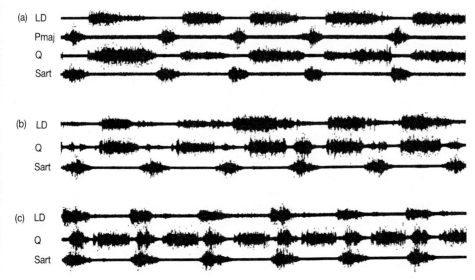

Fig. 6.2   The isolated spinal cord of the cat is able to produce all the stepping patterns or programmes seen in the intact animal, e.g. pacing, trotting. The EMG recording of (a, b) pacing, and (c) trotting seen above were taken from the forelimb and hindlimb of the same side in acute high spinal cats stepping on a treadmill. Pacing and trotting are both examples of alternate gaits where the homologous limbs (forelimbs and hindlimbs) step out of phase. In pacing, the homolateral limbs (hindlimb and forelimb of the same side) are coupled in phase. (a) Activity in the flexor pectoralis major (Pmaj) of the forelimb of the acute high spinal cat coupled with activity in the flexor sartorius (Sart) of the hindlimb. Extensors latissimus dorsi (LD) and quadriceps (Q) of the forelimb and hindlimb are also closely coupled. (b) The same coupling in another experiment. In trotting, the homolateral limbs are coupled out of phase. (c) Activity in extensor LD in the forelimb coupled with activity on flexor Sart in the hindlimb. Reproduced with kind permission from Miller and van der Meché, 1976.

have shown that basic movement patterns of alternating flexion and extension as seen in locomotion are generated by the spinal cord. Isolation of the spinal cord by deafferentation showed that the stepping patterns are also possible without peripheral input. More recent studies (see Grillner, 1981) have supported these earlier ideas with modern physiological measurement techniques, and Miller and van der Meché (1976) were able to show that the movement generator in the isolated spinal cord of the cat is capable of producing all the stepping patterns or programmes that have been identified in the intact cat, for example, pacing and trotting (see Fig. 6.2).

These basic stepping patterns have not so far been demonstrated in acute spinal humans although they are seen in babies as automatic walking, a feature which persists for a few weeks after birth and which is presumed to disappear after descending pathways to the spinal cord have matured. Basic movement patterns may also be a characteristic of spasticity, a situation arising due to partial or complete loss of supraspinal influence on the spinal cord. In spasticity, patients exhibit

mass movement patterns in which a limb is moved in a mass flexion or a mass extension pattern. They are unable to modify the patterns as in the normal human gait pattern or to select specific movements such as the isolated movement of one joint. This suggestion of descending input from the brain controlling and modifying the basic patterns supports the findings from the animal studies which show that descending pathways initiate and modify the basic spinal patterns.

6.5   The effect of descending pathways to the spinal cord

Descending pathways from motor centres in the brain constitute the higher levels of motor control and they exert their influence on the spinal cord in its execution of movement. In animal studies into the neural control of locomotion, it has been shown that descending input from the brain is necessary to switch on basic spinal patterns of locomotion. In studies on spinal cats, although the spinal cord was capable of executing the basic movements independently it was necessary to initiate the movements first either by stimulating cut ends of descending pathways or by the injection of substances such as L-dopa or clonidine (Forssberg and Grillner, 1973; Miller and van der Meché, 1976). These drugs exert their effects on terminals of descending axons from the brain stem that release noradrenaline.

Descending pathways are also able to modify the basic spinal patterns. In the cat, many descending pathways have been found to be phasically active during locomotion, suggesting that in locomotion they may have an effect on the different phases; for example, the lateral vestibulo-spinal tract is active during extension while the rubro-spinal tract is active during flexion (Orlovsky, 1972a, b). However, it would appear that while brain stem pathways such as the vestibulo-spinal tract are able to alter only the intensity of activity in muscle groups during phases of locomotion, cortico-spinal pathways are able to reset the spinal movement generator and alter the pattern of activity. Cortico-spinal pathways may also be responsible for the uncoupling of movement generators at different joints in a limb and a lesion to these pathways would therefore lead to the inability to fractionate movement, i.e. perform flexion at one joint in the limb while another is extending.

Traditionally the descending control from motor centres in the brain, which influences the spinal cord mechanisms in the production of movement, is divided into a pyramidal and an extrapyramidal system. The pyramidal system exerts its influence via the cortico-spinal tracts and the cortico-bulbar tracts. The cortico-spinal tracts form the pyramids as they pass through the medulla and give the system its name. The extrapyramidal system then consists of all other tracts, other than the pyramidal tracts, that influence the spinal cord. The direct cortico-spinal tract or pyramidal system was thought to initiate voluntary movement while the extrapyramidal system was thought to control both voluntary movement and automatic postural adjustments,.

More recently, neuroanatomical and behavioural studies in cats and monkeys (Kuypers, 1973; Lawrence and Kuypers, 1968a, b) have suggested that the descending systems of motor control should be divided into a ventromedial and a dorsolateral division. The ventromedial division includes the tecto-spinal and interstitio-spinal pathways (from the midbrain), the reticulo-spinal pathways, the vestibulo-spinal pathways and the ventral cortico-spinal pathways. The dorsolateral division includes the lateral cortico-spinal pathways, the rubro-spinal pathways and the cortico-bulbar pathways to brain stem nuclei of cranial motor nerves. These ventromedial and dorsolateral divisions are so called because of their relative positions as they pass through the brain stem. They also appear to terminate in the ventral horn of the spinal cord in either a ventromedial position or a dorsolateral position. In this way it would appear that the ventromedial pathways are able to influence, through interneurons, alpha-motoneurons that supply proximal limb muscles and muscles of the trunk, head and neck. Dorsolateral pathways would appear to influence alpha-motoneurons that supply muscles of the distal parts of the limbs (see Fig. 6.3).

In the behavioural studies conducted on Rhesus monkeys by Lawrence and Kuypers (1968a, b) the effects of selected lesions of the pyramidal tracts and descending brain stem pathways were studied. Following lesions of the pyramidal tracts, the monkeys showed limb movements that were lacking in speed and agility. Specially constructed tests showed a lack of individual movements of the fingers and the ability to execute the pinch–grip. Interruption of the ventromedial and dorsolateral brain stem pathways produced two contrasting disturbances. Interruption of the dorsolateral brain stem pathway (the rubro-spinal tract), in combination with pyramidotomy, resulted in an impairment of independent distal extremity movements and an impaired capacity to flex the extended limb. Total limb movements and combined movements of body and limbs were relatively unaffected. Interruption of the ventromedial brain stem pathway resulted in a severe impairment of trunk and proximal limb movements and there was a flexion bias of trunk and limbs. Balance and righting reflexes also seemed to be affected and the animals tended to fall over.

Post mortem studies in humans (Bucy *et al.*, 1964) have supported the view that a pure lesion of the pyramidal tract does not produce a major motor deficit but results in a general reduction in tone and loss of selective movements of distal parts of the limbs. On this basis, it has been concluded that the ventromedial brain stem pathways and the medial cortico-spinal pathway are responsible for the initiation of voluntary movement and of automatic postural adjustments and control of the trunk, head, neck and proximal limbs. The dorsolateral brain stem pathway (the rubro-spinal tract) is

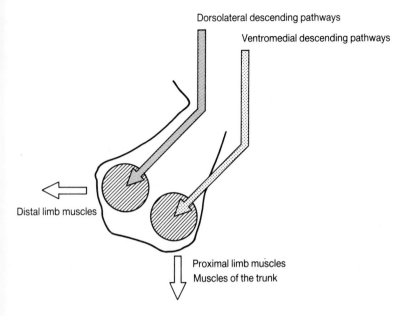

Dorsolateral descending pathways

Ventromedial descending pathways

Distal limb muscles

Proximal limb muscles
Muscles of the trunk

Fig. 6.3 In the ventral horn of the spinal cord, dorsolateral descending pathways terminate preferentially in the dorsolateral region where they influence interneurons and alpha-motoneurons that control distal limb muscles. Ventromedial descending pathways terminate preferentially in the ventromedial region where they influence interneurons and through them alpha-motoneurons that control muscles of the trunk and proximal limb regions.

responsible for control of intrinsic limb movements particularly flexion while the lateral cortico-spinal pathway is only solely responsible for speed and agility of movement and individual movements of the fingers and the pinch–grip. It must be remembered that the rubro-spinal tract which is a major component of the dorsolateral division in cats and also in monkeys is rudimentary in humans and possibly reaches only as far as the upper two segments of the spinal cord (Barr and Kiernan, 1988), although information on this subject is limited and therefore opinions differ. As the cortico-bulbar tract influences the brain stem, the lateral cortico-spinal tract is the major part of the dorsolateral division of descending pathways having influence on the spinal cord in humans.

6.6 Spinal reflex activity and the effect of afferent input from the periphery

Afferent input from the periphery provides feedback to various levels of the CNS in its control of movement. Afferent input to spinal cord level acts as an adjunct to the descending pathways from the brain in their initiation and modification of basic movement patterns. Studies in cats have shown that peripheral input caused by loading of a limb can initiate stepping patterns in the isolated spinal cord and also modify those patterns (see Grillner, 1981). Pearson and Duysens (1976) showed that

prolonging loading on a limb in a mesencephalic cat causes a concomitant prolongation of extensor activity in the limb while the other limbs maintain their phasic activity. The studies have suggested several peripheral receptors as responsible for these effects. They may be due to receptors in muscles, joints or skin but they all appear to be mainly in the proximal regions of the limb. Grillner and Rossignol (1978a) were able to show in experiments with chronic spinal cats that the swing phase could be initiated by extension of the hip joint but the ankle and knee joints did not have the same effect. Anderson *et al.* (1978) also distinguished between hip movements and movements of the knee and ankle in spinal cats. They showed that the frequency of the phasic flexor activity occurring during flexion could be altered by repeated movements of the hip joint into flexion. After deafferentation of the lower part of the limb (ankle and knee region) the frequency of phasic activity in ventral root filaments originally destined for the ankle and knee regions could still be altered by hip movement. As there was no input from the lower regions, movements of the knee and ankle could not be responsible. This initiation and modification of basic spinal patterns by input from proximal regions of the limbs suggests that the input which reaches ventromedial parts of the ventral horn may be able to augment the activity of medial pathways in the intact animal.

It has also been shown that stimulation of peripheral receptors can have different effects depending on the original state of the limb. Cutaneous reflexes from the dorsum of the paw of chronic spinal cats walking on a treadmill appear to enhance the existing state such that if a tactile stimulus is applied during the stance phases then it causes a reinforcement of extension; if applied during the swing phase it reinforces flexion (Forssberg *et al.*, 1975). This effect, called 'phase-dependent reflex reversal' by Forssberg and his colleagues was also demonstrated in the response to a contralateral stimulus (Grillner and Rossignol, 1978b; Rossignol and Gautier, 1980). This supported the observations of Magnus (1909) who observed that in chronic spinal dogs the initial position of a limb could determine its response to a knee tap applied to the contralateral limb, and also the observation of von Uexkull (1904) on the brittlestar. Rossignol and Gautier (1980) suggested that the evidence from their observations indicated that there are pathways to both flexors and extensors from cutaneous receptors. They also suggested that the interpretation by Magnus (1910) that the crossed reflex response is directed towards the muscle which is most stretched is not wholly true as in their observations the extensor responses appear even after deafferentiation. Grillner and Rossignol (1978b) also suggest that the response does not depend upon the state of stretch of the responding muscles as after tenotomy, the retracted muscles of an antagonistic pair respond at the same time as their synergists at other joints which are stretched or relaxed during manipulation of the whole limb. Present knowledge of the integration of reflex pathways in the spinal cord and the sharing of interneurons and motorneurons by different reflex pathways could mean that the peripheral signals are inducing the appropriate response by raising the excitability of a specific neuronal pool or by inhibiting activity in another.

Lundberg (1979) also considered the different effects that may occur when flexor reflex afferents (FRA) are stimulated. Flexor reflex afferents are group II and III afferents arising in muscle, joint and skin receptors and are traditionally thought to respond to noxious stimuli only and to result in a flexion withdrawal reflex. Lundberg, however, suggested that the FRA can be stimulated by movement alone. Anden *et al.* (1966) have shown in the acute spinal cat that stimulation of the FRA produces a short-latency reflex that causes ipsilateral limb flexion and a contralateral limb exten-

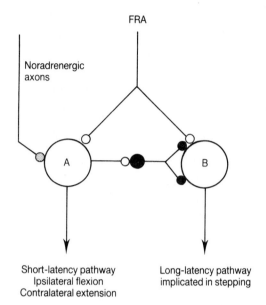

Fig. 6.4 In the acute spinal cat, stimulation of the flexor reflex afferents (FRA) produces a short-latency reflex that causes ipsilateral limb flexion and a contralateral limb extension, but after injection of dopa long-latency reflexes appear. Lundberg (1979) suggests that in the intact animal the short-latency pathway is inhibited by descending noradrenergic terminals thus releasing the long-latency pathway from inhibition as shown above. Combined stimulation of ipsilateral and contralateral FRA in the acute spinal cat injected with dopa (i.e. with the long-latency pathway disinhibited) reveals a reciprocal organization in that either flexors or extensors are activated. This leads to the suggestion that long-latency pathways may play a role in stepping. The short latency reflexes may also be seen in spinal humans as the heightened flexor withdrawal reflex. The inhibition of the long-latency pathway in this situation could lead to a difficulty in initiating basic spinal patterns such as those of stepping as seen in patients with spasticity.

sion, but after injection of dopa long-latency reflexes appear. Lundberg suggested that the short-latency reflex inhibits the long-latency reflex. Dopa causes a transmitter release from descending nor-adrenergic pathways which inhibit the short-latency reflex so that the long-latency reflex is released from its inhibitory control (see Fig. 6.4). Combined stimulation of ipsilateral and contralateral FRA in the acute spinal cat injected with dopa intravenously reveals a reciprocal organization in that either flexor or extensor motorneurons are activated (Jankowska *et al.*, 1967). Lundberg therefore suggested that the long-latency FRA pathway may play a part in inducing the basic spinal patterns of flexion and extension of locomotion. If this is true and if the same situation exists in humans then the active flexion withdrawal reflex often seen in patients with spasticity could be due to lack of inhibition of the short-latency FRA pathway caused by damage to descending tracts. A lack of inhibition of the short-latency pathway would then lead to an inhibition by this pathway of the long-latency pathway. This would lead to a difficulty in initiating basic spinal patterns – a characteristic of spasticity.

The role of spinal reflex activity in supporting and facilitating movement has become evident with the many studies of reflex activity occurring due to the stimulation of peripheral receptors such as the muscle spindle, the golgi tendon organs and other muscle, joint and cutaneous receptors (for an extensive review see Rothwell, 1987). Evidence from these studies has pointed to a wide convergence onto interneurons within the spinal cord showing that many reflex pathways share common interneurons. Convergent input onto interneurons may be from descending input from the brain as well as from the peripheral receptors and the knowledge of integration of spinal reflex pathways has increased the understanding of movement control. Movement may result from activity in several reflex and voluntary pathways causing firing of interneurons through spatial summation but in many situations it may be necessary to inhibit or modulate activity in one pathway while leaving other pathways open.

Modulation of transmission in spinal reflex pathways may be achieved through a postsynaptic inhibition of interneurons within the pathways or through a presynaptic inhibition of one or more of the afferent fibres converging onto the interneurons. Presynaptic inhibition is caused by a depolarization of afferent fibres at their presynaptic site leading to a decrease in the amount of transmitter substance released into the synaptic cleft by an action potential travelling along the afferent fibre. This therefore leads to a reduction in the size of the postsynaptic potential produced in the postsynaptic neuron. However, the ability of other afferent terminals on the same postsynaptic neuron to produce postsynaptic potentials is unaltered. Most dorsal root fibres can presynaptically inhibit themselves (see Rothwell, 1987), the inhibition occurring through the stimulation of an interneuron which then depolarizes the dorsal root fibre. It is possible that the interneuron may be switched on by the action of descending fibres as well as by peripheral afferent fibres themselves and in this way presynaptic inhibition would be able to modulate or 'gate' incoming sensory information. Incoming painful stimuli can be modulated by the stimulation of descending tracts, notably the raphe spinal tract and also by stimulation of peripheral afferent fibres, notably the large diameter group I fibres. This inhibition appears to be due to presynaptic as well as postsynaptic effects (Wall, 1989).

It has been suggested that the inhibition of short-latency flexor reflexes by activity in noradrenergic terminals in the spinal cord occurs through a process of supraspinal presynaptic inhibition but that a segmental presynaptic inhibition in which the FRA control their own activity through a negative feedback mechanism may also play a part (Lundberg, 1979). The absence or reduction of supraspinal inhibition both presynaptic as well as postsynaptic, may be the main cause of the increase in muscle tone and hyperflexia seen in patients with spasticity (see Burke, 1980, 1983; and also Chapter 9). Recent studies in chronic spinal humans have shown that the administration of oral clonidine causes a subjective decrease in spinal reflex activity and an increase in vibratory inhibition of the H-reflex, indicating a restoration of presynaptic inhibition due to activity in noradrenergic terminals (Nance *et al.*, 1990). It may be possible in humans to induce a segmental presynaptic inhibition through manipulation of afferent stimuli as in the control of pain through stimulation of large diameter afferents (as in acupuncture, transcutaneous electrical nerve stimulation). Observations in spastic humans have suggested that it is possible to reduce muscle tone through the alteration of proximal limb positions (Bobath, 1990) although no experimental studies to investigate the effect on vibratory inhibition of the H-reflex and therefore on presynaptic inhibition have been carried out.

6.7 The role of higher centres of motor control

The cortical areas in the precentral and postcentral gyri are referred to as the motorsensory cortex (Ms) and the sensorimotor cortex (Sm) because of their predominant involvement in motor or sensory activities. The precentral gyrus (Brodmann's area 4) initiates movement by directing the spinal cord in its activities. Electrical stimulation of area 4 causes contraction of specific muscles on the opposite side of the body and damage to area 4 causes a flaccid paralysis. Area 4 receives input mainly from the premotor area (area 6), the postcentral gyrus (the Sm) and the posterior division of the ventral lateral thalamic nucleus (VLp), which itself receives input from the cerebellum. This means that area 4 is able to initiate movement at the direction of the premotor area and adjust that movement at the direction of the cerebellum. Sensory input can also initiate activity in area 4 cells due to long-loop reflexes and a study in monkeys (Evarts and Tanji, 1976) suggests that this long-loop reflex activity through the Sm can be controlled by the premotor cortex (see Cheney, 1985, for review).

While area 4 directs the spinal cord in its activities, the premotor area (area 6) directs area 4 in its activities. The premotor area receives input partly via the corpus striatum and the anterior division of the ventral lateral thalamic nucleus (VLa), from the prefrontal cortex where ideas and the motivation for movement are generated and also from sensory association areas of the cortex. The premotor area is thought to be concerned with the elaboration or building up of programmes for learned skilled movement, information on which can then be sent to the Ms. In normal movement the Ms rarely initiates the contraction of a single muscle but initiates a programme or pattern of activity, information on which is received from the other higher centres such as the premotor area. For this reason area 4 is often said to be concerned not with muscle contraction but with patterns of movement. These patterns are modifications of the basic spinal patterns. The premotor area also bypasses area 4 to project to the spinal cord both directly via the cortico-spinal fibres and indirectly via the brain stem.

The corpus striatum, which projects to the premotor cortex, receives its input from a wide area of the cerebral cortex, particularly from the frontal and parietal lobes, and by sending information to the premotor area it is able to help in the control of movement. The precise function of the basal ganglia, of which the corpus striatum forms the major part, is unknown but the corpus striatum is able to affect output from the Ms and also affect the spinal cord, both through its connections with the premotor area. Output from the premotor area to the spinal cord via the brain stem is thought to be concerned with the control of proximal regions of the limbs and may be a way in which output from the corpus striatum can control background postural adjustment. The basal ganglia are also thought to help in the regulation of muscle tone and lesions of the basal ganglia invariably lead to disturbances in muscle tone causing either involuntary movements due to fluctuating tone or akinesia due to excessive tone.

The cerebellum is also an important organ in the control of movement. It can be divided into three regions according to its phylogenetic development: the archicerebellum, the paleocerebellum and the neocerebellum (see Barr and Kiernan, 1988). The archicerebellum has reciprocal connections with brain stem areas concerned with balance and it is concerned with the regulation of balance and righting reactions. The paleocerebellum and the neocerebellum are concerned with movement control, in particular, with the coordination of movement. Without cerebellar influence movement is jerky and inaccurate. The paleocerebellum and the neocerebellum receive information from the Ms on intended movement and also receive information from the spinal cord on the actual movement that has taken place. The cerebellum is able to bring about an adjustment of the output from the Ms to make the movement more accurate. In humans where the neocerebellum is most developed it is now also thought to have a role in motor learning (see Ghez and Fahn, 1985).

6.8 Influencing movement through manipulation of peripheral input

In the short-term, stimulation of peripheral receptors has been shown to influence motor output from the spinal cord. This influence is exerted at several levels of the neuraxis but it is particularly powerful in its effect at spinal cord level. In initiating and modifying basic spinal patterns, peripheral input is bypassing the Ms and therefore through its direct effect on the spinal cord provides a third parallel system (see Section 6.2 and Fig. 6.1) in combination with the pathways from the Ms and the brain stem. Higher centres of motor control are able to influence the Ms and the brain stem in their effect on the spinal cord and the Ms can influence the brain stem. As described above, there is also evidence for the modulation of peripheral input or its effects on spinal reflex activity by higher centres, notably by the sensorimotor cortex via cortico-spinal fibres and by the brain stem. This controlling effect may be either facilitatory or inhibitory and the inhibition is probably both presynaptic and postsynaptic.

In normal intact humans these three parallel systems, periphery, brain stem and motorsensory cortex, affect the spinal cord together so the peripheral input acts as an adjunct to the more sophisticated control exerted through the Ms. Various spinal reflex actions help to support the actions of the motorsensory cortex while the sensorimotor cortex and the brain stem modulate the effects of peripheral input.

The fact that peripheral input supports cortical control has been exploited in rehabilitation of brain-damaged patients who have lost elements of descending control from the Ms. Stimulation of cutaneous afferents during movement helps to reinforce both alpha- and gamma-motoneuron activity in underlying muscles (Eldred and Hagbarth, 1954) and increases Ib inhibition of more distant muscles (Pierrot-Deseilligny *et al.*, 1981a) and this has led to the use of cutaneous input to facilitate movement. Also Ia afferent input from a contracting muscle will facilitate alpha efferent activity to other muscles or muscle groups. This idea of Ia afferent overflow to more distant muscles was first postulated by Eccles and Lundberg in 1958 from studies in the cat and it has been used to facilitate the contraction of weak muscle groups by first initiating a contraction of a stronger group. Recent studes (Pierrot-Deseilligny *et al.*, 1981b; Forget *et al.*, 1989) have confirmed this effect in humans by demonstrating the facilitation of the quadriceps H-reflex by the stimulation of group I afferents from pretibial flexors both while the quadriceps is at rest and during a voluntary contraction. However, many other muscle groups need investigating before a comprehensive pattern of facilitation can be drawn up.

The use of peripheral input through movement of proximal limb regions has also been used to facilitate normal muscle tone and fractionated movement by aiding in the initiation and modification of basic spinal patterns of movement. It seems possible that the input is gating some spinal cord pathways while allowing transmission in others. However, these many spinal circuits are not 'hard-wired' and activity in a circuit will lead to the reinforcement of that circuit. Movement itself therefore provides the correct sensory input to facilitate and reinforce itself by the strengthening of synaptic 'sets' (see Chapter 4). This means that normal movement patterns reinforce normal movement patterns in the long-term through the strengthening of synaptic pathways involved in the movements. A knowledge of the ways on which normal movement can be facilitated through the manipulation of peripheral input should therefore help in the long-term rehabilitation of patients with movement disorders. This topic will be explored further in Chapter 9.

References

Anden, N. E., Jukes, M. G. M., Lundberg, A. and Viklicky, L. (1966). The effect of dopa on the spinal cord. 1. Influence on transmission from primary afferents. *Acta Physiologica Scandinavica* **67**: 373–86.

Anderson, O., Grillner, S., Lindquist, M. and Zomlefer, M. (1978) Peripheral control of the spinal pattern generators for locomotion in the cat. *Brain Research* **150**: 625–30.

Barr, M. L. and Kiernan, J. A. (1988) *The Human Nervous System.* Philadelphia: Lippincott.

Bobath, B. (1990) *Adult Hemiplegia: Evaluation and Treatment.* London: Heinemann.

Brown, T. G. (1911) The intrinsic factor in the act of progression in the mammal. *Proceedings of the Royal Society* **B84**: 308–19.

Bucy, P. C., Kephinger, J. E. and Siqueira, E. B. (1964) Destruction of the pyramidal tract in man. *Journal of Neurosurgery* **21**: 385–98.

Burke, D. (1980) A reassessment of the muscle spindle contribution to muscle tone in normal and spastic man. In: Feldman, R. G., Young, R. R. and Koella, W. P., eds. *Spasticity: Disordered Motor Control.* Chicago: Year Book Medical Publications, pp. 261–78.

Burke, D. (1983) Critical examination of the case for or against fusimotor involvement in disorders of muscle tone. In: Desmedt, J. E., ed. *Motor Control Mechanisms in Health and Disease. Advances in Neurology.* Volume 39. New York: Raven Press, pp. 133–50.

Cheney, P. D. (1985) The role of the cerebral cortex in voluntary movement: a review. *Physical Therapy* **65**: 624–35.

Eccles, E. and Lundberg, A. (1958) Integrative patterns of Ia synaptic actions on motorneurones of hip and knee muscles. *Journal of Physiology* **144**: 271–98.

Eldred, E. and Hagbarth, K-E. (1954) Facilitation and inhibition of gamma efferents by stimulation of certain skin areas. *Journal of Neurophysiology* **17**: 59–65.

Evarts, E. V. and Tanji, J. (1976) Reflex and intended responses in motor cortex pyramidal tract neurones of monkey. *Journal of Neurophysiology* **37**: 1069–80.

Forget, R., Hultborn, H., Meunier, S., Pantieri, R. and Pierrot-Deseilligny, E. (1989) Facilitation of quadriceps motorneurones by group I afferents from pretibial flexors in man. 2. Changes occurring during voluntary contractions. *Experimental Brain Research* **78**: 21–7.

Forssberg, H. and Grillner, S. (1973) The locomotion of the acute spinal cat injected with clonidine i.v. *Brain Research* **50**: 184–6.

Forssberg, H., Grillner, S. and Rossignol, S. (1975) Phase dependent reflex reversal during walking in chronic spinal cats. *Brain Research* **85**: 103–7.

Ghez, C. (1985) Introduction to the motor systems. In Kandel, E. R. and Schwartz, J. H., eds. *Principles of Neural Science.* Part VI: *Motor Systems of the Brain: Reflex and Voluntary Control of Movement.* New York: Elsevier, pp. 429–42.

Ghez, C. and Fahn, S. (1985) The cerebellum. In Kandel, E. R. and Schwartz, J. H., eds. *Principles of Neural Science*. Part VI: *Motor Systems of the Brain: Reflex and Voluntary Control of Movement*. New York: Elsevier, pp. 502–22.

Grillner, S. (1981) Control of locomotion in bipedes, tetrapodes and fish. In Brooks, V., ed. *Handbook of Physiology*. Volume III, Section I: *The Nervous System, II. Motor Control*. Baltimore: American Physiological Society, Waverley Press, 1179–1236.

Grillner, S. and Rossignol, S. (1978a) On the initiation of the swing phase of locomotion in chronic spinal cats. *Brain Research* **146**: 269–77.

Grillner, S. and Rossignol, S. (1978b) Contralateral reflex reversal controlled by limb position in the acute spinal cat injected with clonidine i.v. *Brain Research* **144**: 411-4.

Illingworth, R. S. (1987) *The Development of the Infant and Young Child: Normal and Abnormal*. Edinburgh: Churchill Livingstone.

Jackson, J. H. (1884) Croonian lectures on the evolution and dissolution of the nervous system. *Lancet* **i**: 555–8.

Jankowska, E., Jukes, M. G. M., Lund, S. and Lundberg, A. (1967) The effect of dopa on the spinal cord. 5. Reciprocal organization of pathways transmitting excitatory action to alpha motorneurons of flexors and extensors. *Acta Physiologica Scandinavica* **70**: 369-88.

Kuypers, H. G. J. M. (1973) The anatomical organization of the descending pathways and their contribution to motor control especially in primates. In Desmedt, J. E., ed. *New Developments in EMG and Clinical Neurophysiology*. Volume 3. Basel: Karger, pp. 38–68.

Lawrence, D. G. and Kuypers, H. G. J. M. (1968a) The functional organization of the motor systems in the monkey. 1. The effect of bilateral pyramidal lesions. *Brain* **91**: 1–14.

Lawrence, D. G. and Kuypers, H. G. J. M. (1968b) The functional organization of the motor systems in the monkey. 2. The effects of lesions of the descending brainstem pathways. *Brain* **91**: 15–33.

Lundberg, A. (1979) Multisensory control of spinal reflex pathways. *Progress in Brain Research* **50**: 11–28.

Magnus, R. (1909) Regelung der bewegungen durch das zentralnervensystem. Mitteilung I. *Pflugers Arch. Ges. Physiol.* **130**: 219–52.

Magnus, R. (1910) Regelung der bewegungen durch das zentralnervensystem. Mitteilung III. *Pflugers Archiv fur die Gesamte Physiologie des Menschen und der Tiere* **134**: 545–83.

Miller, S. and van der Meché, F. G. A. (1976) Co-ordinated stepping of all four limbs in the high spinal cat. *Brain Research* **109**: 395–8.

Nance, P. W., Shears, A. H. and Nance, D. M. (1990) Reflex changes induced by clonidine in spinal cord injured patients. *Paraplegia* **27**: 296–301.

Orlovsky, G. N. (1972a) Activity of vestibulospinal neurones during locomotion. *Brain Research* **46**: 85-98.

Orlovsky, G. N. (1972b) Activity of rubrospinal neurones during locomotion. *Brain Research* **46**: 99–112.

Pearson, K. G. and Duysens, J. (1976) Function of segmental reflexes in the control of stepping in cockroaches and cats. In Herman, R. M., Grillner, S., Stein, P. S. G. and Stuart, D. G., eds. *Neural Control of Locomotion*. New York: Plenum Press, pp. 519–35.

Pierrot-Deseilligny, E., Bergego, C., Katz, R. *et al.* (1981a) Cutaneous depression of Ib reflex pathways to motorneurones in man. *Experimental Brain Research* **42**: 351–61.

Pierrot-Deseilligny, E., Morin, C., Bergego, C. and Tankov, N. (1981b) Pattern of group I fibre projections from ankle flexor and extensor muscles in man. *Experimental Brain Research* **42**: 337–50.

Rossignol, S. and Gautier L. (1980) Reversal of contralateral limb reflexes. *Proceedings of the International Union of the Physiological Sciences* **13**: 639.

Rothwell, J. C. (1987) *Control of Human Voluntary Movement*. London: Croom Helm.

Sherrington, C. S. (1910) Flexion-reflex of the limb, crossed extension-reflex and reflex stepping and standing. *Journal of Physiology* **40**: 28–121.

Uexkull, J. von (1904) Die ersten ursachen des rythmus in der tierreihe. *Ergebrnsse der Physiologie* **3**: 1–11.

Wall, P. D. (1989) The dorsal horn. In Wall, P. D. and Melzack, R. eds. *Textbook of Pain*. Edinburgh: Churchill Livingstone, pp. 102–11.

Chapter 7

The plasticity of skeletal muscle

7.1 Muscle FORM and muscle FUNCTION. The concept of FORMFUNCTION

Skeletal muscle is one of the most plastic tissues in the human body. This plasticity is shown by a muscle's liability to change. With a stability of the conditions influencing a skeletal muscle there is a stability also of the form of the fibres which comprise it and of the mechanical action they generate. When change is imposed on the mechanical action of this muscle it is surprisingly mutable. This is seen easily as change in muscle form, but changes in muscle function can be seen also. It is here that the concept of FORMFUNCTION is valuable. We are looking for a different form of bioengineering which does not overemphasize BIOENGINEER-ING by giving equal attention to both roots of the word. On the other hand bioENGINEERING considered the mechanical components of muscles acting about the joints of the body behaving as a system of levers. It is almost as though the living nature of skeletal muscle was being overlooked, or at the best diminished. We should aim for a better balance and, at the risk of an opposing overattention, we will consider BIOengineering where the engineering is one in which the molecular machines and their controls are tuned and turned to serve the purpose of rehabilitation.

When approaching a study of such a biologically fundamental process as plastic adaptation, it is better not to stay with simple and descriptive labels. We must develop an approach to the subject at the level of the macromolecule. The form of a skeletal muscle, to take an example from an earlier anatomy, was often described pictorially by its Latin name. *Gastrocnemius*, for instance, is a muscle of the leg (*kneme*) which bellies (*gastro-*), as a sail bellies. The muscle *tibialis anterior* is associated anatomically with the *tibia*, a bone so called because it resembles a musical pipe or flute.

Some muscles are classified as extensors, where extension can be defined exactly as a movement in the sagittal plane of the body which returns a body part back to its natural anatomical position and beyond it (Tyldesley and Grieve, 1989). Some muscles are involved in the tonic action of the postural control system, whereas others are phasic in their pattern of activity and the timing of their mechanical role in the systems of motor control.

Alternatively, muscles may be classified in the general terms of their spurt or shunt mechanical action (MacConnail and Basmajian, 1969). Examples of primarily spurt muscles are given as *biceps brachii* acting with *brachialis* upon the elbow joint, and of a shunt muscle as *brachioradialis* acting upon the same joint. Should they be reversed functionally, then the spurt muscle will become a shunt muscle and conversely. As the authors make clear, when the foot is taken off the ground then the hamstring muscles (*biceps femoris, semitendinosus* and *semimembranosus*) are spurt muscles to the knee joint and shunt extensors to the hip. But they become shunt flexors to the knee and spurt extensors to the hip when the foot is placed back upon the ground and kept there.

The preceding examples already allow us to question the adequacy of considering separately the FORM and FUNCTION of a skeletal muscle. A totally different approach, but one which allows the concept of a plastic adaptation to develop, comes from a consideration of the embryogenesis of skeletal muscle (Vrbová *et al.*, 1978; Spielholz, 1982).

We should first set the stage upon which the plastic adaptation of skeletal muscle is performed. In the embryo, during the stages of myogenesis, the undifferentiated cells which are destined to become fibres of skeletal muscle are contained in the middle sheet of developing cells: the mesoderm (Fig. 7.1).

The premyoblasts under a light microscope are seen to be a loose mass of individual mononuclear cells. Only some of these cells are myogenic stem cells, whilst others will become fibroblasts which, with subsequent development, will form the connective tissue of the developing skeletal muscle. During this early stage of gestation, the truly myogenic cells are replicating under a non-muscle genetic programme.

Later in gestation, a population of myoblasts fuse to form multinucleated myotubes. Although at this stage, the cross-striations of skeletal muscle are not visible under a light microscope, an electron microscope reveals early signs of the synthesis of the molecules defining myofibrils. During embryonic development muscle cells are nowhere near maturity. Myoblasts continue to leave the proliferative phase of early development and fuse to myotubes and form muscle fibres.

Myotube diameters increase as a continuation of development. They synthesize myofibrils, and other sarcoplasmic constituents (for example, the network of the sarcoplasmic reticulum and the T-tubule systems). Even in the human neonate, skeletal muscle development is incomplete. It is at these stages of late gestation and during the early neonatal period of growth that the muscle fibres show the pluripotentiality of later development and respond genetically to extrinsic factors of control.

In Fig. 7.2, all of the developing muscular system is simplified to a circular cell containing a nucleus. Gene expression, the relative magnitude of which is represented by the broadness of the vertically oriented arrow, can be modified by factors external, or extrinsic, to the cells. Therapists are, of course, important extrinsic factors where the application of the elements of neuromuscular plasticity is concerned. That factor is indicated diagrammatically by the breadth of the arrow directed at the nuclei.

The preceding detail of the stages in the embryological development of skeletal muscle was presented as an attempt to make clear that the widening of the range of motor activity can be a major factor in determining the phenotype of mature muscle fibres.

These extrinsic factors will be exerted subsequently upon skeletal muscle, and they will influence strongly the direction of plastic adaptation by the skeletomotor system. The factors are of great importance during the response of the system to carefully directed procedures of physical conditioning and training such as seen during the development of an élite athlete. The performance of an athlete, to take just one end of the spectrum of physical performance, is determined in part by the force–velocity relationship developed by an active muscle. In that relationship, as the velocity

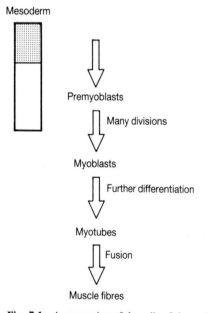

Fig. 7.1 A proportion of the cells of the embryonic myoderm (shaded, upper left) is the origin of striated muscle. Successive division and differentiation gives rise to myotubes which fuse end-to-end to produce striated muscle fibres. Control of cell development is initially under a non-muscle genetic programme but the muscle fibre produced eventually is under an external or exogenous control. Fully effective rehabilitation requires an understanding and an application of this control.

Motor development

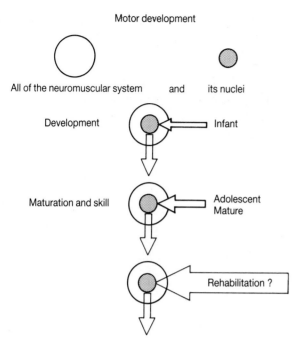

Fig. 7.2 All of the cells of the neuromuscular system and their nuclei are represented diagrammatically by the two circles. Gene expression, naturally and exogenously controlled, is represented, respectively, by the vertical and horizontal arrows. Exogenous control modulates gene expression and becomes specifically effective during rehabilitation. Until the professions responsible gain insight, the full effectiveness of rehabilitation will be delayed in its development.

of shortening in a muscle increases, the force it is able to apply decreases. It is appropriate here to offer a reminder that skeletal muscle stopped 'contracting' very early in an elementary education in the basic sciences. We should review therefore the elements of the mechanical actions of skeletal muscle (Fig. 7.3). A muscle must be thought of as opposing the force applied to the body from outside: the world force of the external force. It does so by generating muscular force. When the muscular force is superior to the external force the system acts *concentrically* and the two ends of the muscle approach the midpoint: in that condition and only in that condition does the muscle contract. When the external force is superior to the muscle force, the muscle although active lengthens: the system acts *eccentrically* and the two ends of the muscle move away from the middle. When both muscle force and external force are equal, there is no

change in muscle length and the system acts *isometrically*.

It is important not to confuse the speed of development of these forms of mechanical action with the speed of movement of the body parts controlled by that action. They are not necessarily the same.

Two legs of a patient moving during locomotion, for example, describe an angular arc and may be moving through it at the same speed, but where one leg has a greater physical mass, the greater, per unit of time, must be the muscular force generated by it to move the 'heavier' leg. The muscles which move the 'heavier' leg must develop action at a greater rate, even though both legs have identical velocities of movement.

Slowing down the speed of development of muscular action enables a patient to develop more force. This is true for both the development of concentric action and during the development of isometric action when the two ends of the muscle are prevented from moving in relation to the midpoint, and its length remains unchanging. When the action of the muscle is eccentric the force developed by the muscle is directly proportional to the velocity at which the lengthening takes place.

The word *strength* is often used incorrectly. Are

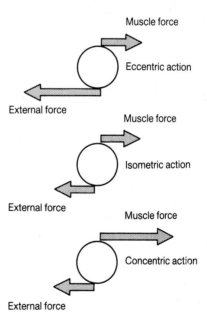

Fig. 7.3 There is a mutual dependence between the motor effect of skeletal muscle and the molecules it contains. Its action in developing eccentric, isometric and concentric force comes also within the range of motor rehabilitation.

you implying, for example, that a skeletal muscle has the strength to move a body part, or do you mean that it has the strength to hold a body part in correct alignment with other parts? A dictionary could define strength as 'the capacity for exertion or endurance', a definition which summarizes well one description of the types of activity which determine the phenotype of skeletal muscle fibres (Pette and Vrbová, 1985).

Skeletal muscle, as it is considered here, is an exceedingly dynamic structure. By that remark we mean being more dynamic than, simply, in its mechanical role. 'Dynamic' concerns in addition the equilibrium of its molecular components (see page 42).

A useful application of the concepts derived from the macromolecular approach to skeletal muscle structure can be applied to the simple equations of muscular action which describe muscular power:

$$\text{Power} = \text{Work/Time} = \text{Force} \times \text{Distance/Time} = \text{Force} \times \text{Velocity}$$

The form of skeletal muscle can be seen to depend therefore upon the functions enforced by the circumstances of its early natural growth and subsequent development. Similarly, an increasing range of functions of the skeletal muscle is *enabled* as the form of the muscle fibres responds by adaptation. So, out of the system, a point within the potential of skeletal muscle can be made actual (Fig. 7.4) by natural procedures of development, and also by an intentionally planned and directed therapy of rehabilitation. Figure 7.4 shows, diagrammatically, how the actual state of skeletal muscle (vertically stippled arrow) and the consequent states

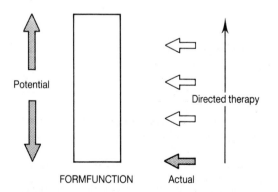

Fig. 7.4 The range of potential of muscle is a factor of its genome. The choice, within this range, is obtained by expressing a phenotype and is accessible by a directed therapy.

as therapy moves actuality (unfilled arrows) in response to an intentional direction by the therapist.

7.2 Adaptation of skeletal muscle during natural development and during therapy

Any discussion of skeletal muscle as an organ in isolation is an unjustifiable abstraction. The pools of motoneurons innervating the muscle, and which employ its muscle units as mechanical transducer of effect, must be brought into a perspective.

Skeletal muscle is the terminal effector located as the end of the 'common final pathway' of the systems of motor control (Sherrington, 1904). The state of skeletal muscle fibres depends upon connection with motor axon terminals, and to some extent the soma (cell body) of the motoneuron depends in turn upon connection with adequate muscles fibres. The scientific aspects of the subject are discussed by Vrbová *et al.* (1978). Price (1974) introduces a more general discussion of how the periphery of the muscular system influences the centrally situated spinal motoneurons.

In the late foetus, the most abundant protein of striated muscle, myosin, has a unique form. The later striated muscle proteins are similar in molecular form to adult fast-twitch muscles (Salmons and Henrikson, 1981). At this point we must examine the criteria for placing motor units into specific types.

7.3 Classifications of motor units

All human striated muscle (with the exception of extraocular muscle, the small muscles of the inner ear and some striated muscle of the oesophagus) is of the twitch type. Muscle fibres are focally innervated by terminal branches of motor axons. The connection is made through nerve-to-muscle synapses or motor endplates, and a single motoneuron innervates many skeletal muscle fibres (the number of muscle fibres innervated by a single motoneuron as its axon branches is referred to as its *innervation ratio*). In general, the smaller the ratio, the greater the delicacy of muscle action and the finer the motor control applied to it. Conversely, coarse muscular action and its control are applied through a motor unit with a large innervation ratio.

Numerically, the innervation ratio can vary from less than 5 to 3000 or over. Motoneurons occupy the anterior horn of the spinal cord (as Rexed lamina- or spinal nucleus-IX) and form the cranial motor nuclei of the brain stem. Those with a relatively small cell body (soma) diameter innervate a muscle unit comprised of mechanically slow-twitch muscle fibres. Large soma diameter motoneurons innervate a muscle unit with mechanically fast-twitch characteristics.

Each motoneuron not only determines the mechanical response of its muscle unit, but it also controls the physiological and biochemical properties of the muscle fibres. A broad classification of motor units introduces three types:

1. **S**-type motor units which are mechanically **S**low and contain muscle which is **S**low to fatigue, for example, in *soleus*.

2. **FF** types which are mechanically **F**ast and the muscles is **F**ast to develop fatigue, for example, in *tibialis anterior*.

3. **FR** types which are mechanically **F**ast and the muscle is more **R**esistant to fatigue, for example, in *gastrocnemius*.

Introducing some features of the metabolism of the muscle fibres in each type can further define the classification.

(a) **SO** (type I) motor units which are mechanically **S**low with an **O**xidative metabolism.
(b) **FG** (type II) motor units which are mechanically **F**ast with a **G**lycolytic metabolism.
(c) **FOG** motor units which are mechanically **F**ast with an **O**xidative capacity which almost matches the **G**lycolytic capacity.

This form of classification relates almost completely to the earlier classifications of skeletal muscle into RED (**SO**), WHITE (**FG**) and INTERMEDIATE (**FOG**).

A useful attempt at reduction in the complexity of this muscle fibre adopted a numerical description of the typing and led to the type I, IIA, IIB (with type IIAB as a possible intermediary) and IIC classification. This classification which allows for muscle fibre types that are not covered by the functional and biochemical categories described above is handled with clarity by English and Wolf (1982). Essentially, type I muscle fibres cover a twitch mechanical action which develops force slowly to reach its peak, and relaxes the developed force slowly as well. Type II muscle fibres develop

a twitch of force quickly and relax it similarly. Type I muscle fibres are slow to fatigue but type II muscle fibres fatigue rapidly. The additional types accommodate muscle fibre actions which do not fit easily into the less comprehensive classification. We feel that it not only presents a broader range of muscle fibre characteristics but justifies also the expression FORMFUNCTION and underlines the dynamic mutability of the motor unit that we are emphasizing in this book.

The full detail of the complexity is discussed by Guba (1981) where the advantages and limitations of the wealth of molecular detail are both set out clearly. An important demonstration of the anatomical properties of the distribution of the muscle unit of a single motor unit followed the application of the glycogen depletion technique (Kugelberg and Edström, 1968). In this technique single motoneurons were stimulated electrically either after impalement in the spinal cord by micropette or following electrical stimulation of a tiny bundle dissected from a ventral root which contained the motor axon of a single motoneuron. Stimulation, by either method, was continued until the stimulated muscle unit was depleted of its glycogen. A comparative histochemical reaction (PAS reaction) was then employed to stain the muscle fibres for microscopic study, and muscle fibres using glycogen could be distinguished from those surrounding them in the anatomical muscle. By using reactions to reveal different metabolic pathways an advance was made into the ability to visualize histochemically, within an anatomical muscle, the distribution of single muscle fibres of different motor units (Burke *et al.*, 1974). These histochemical techniques are discussed, both specifically and in general, by Vrbová *et al.* (1978) and English and Wolf (1982).

7.4 The motor innervation of skeletal muscle

Outgrowth occurs from the embryonic cells developing during neurogenesis of the spinal cord of vertebrates. Some of the developing neurons establish contact with simultaneously developing skeletal muscle (Section 7.1 above).

It is at this point of the discussion of neuromuscular plasticity that care must be taken to separate the careful studies on laboratory animal preparations, which have yielded important scientific detail, from the controlled clinical studies developed from the laboratory work and which have been applied to human rehabilitation.

Most active developing motoneurons are believed to establish a form of contact with skeletal muscle. The more active neurons are successful in establishing functional connection with developing skeletal muscle fibres. Less active neurons do not make effective connection with the muscle fibres of the periphery, and having failed to do so, they die.

As the muscle fibres themselves develop, the exploring motoneurons can make contact with several of them, whereupon a state of polyneuronal innervation is established. Ingrowing axons and the skeletal muscle fibres, respectively, release and are sensitive to acetylcholine. The skeletal muscle, immature at this early stage, has a widely distributed chemosensitivity to acetylcholine over its surface membrane. Following effective innervation, there is a migration of the membrane receptors for acetylcholine within the muscle fibre membrane when they become localized as the subneural apparatus of a motor endplate.

As soon as the endplates become visible microscopically, the membrane outside the point of contact with the nerve terminal (the extrajunctional membrane) becomes desensitized and unresponsive to acetylcholine. The developing motor controls at this stage of innervation limit the degree of polyneuronal innervation by eliminating progressively those neuromuscular junctions which are the least effective. This continuous 'remodelling' of the motor innervation of skeletal muscle fibres is described by Vrbová *et al.* (1989). The essential point here of the 'remodelling' is that the effectiveness and indeed the purposefulness of a developing motor control can in some way 'fine tune' the terminal motor innervation.

The process of elimination of excess motor terminals on the maturing muscle fibre has to be dependent on the activity of the postsynaptic membrane (that is, of the skeletal muscle fibre). The smaller and most probably the least effective of the neuromuscular terminal structures are preferentially eliminated because of the electrical effect of K^+, released as a consequence of muscle fibre activity. This ion activates in turn voltage-dependent Ca^{2+} channels in the nerve terminals. Whereupon, the Ca^{2+} entering the endplate activates neutral protease (CANP, see Chapter 1, Section 1.6). This is followed by an enzymatic digestion of the cyto-

skeletal elements of the neuromuscular terminal which is believed to cause the removal of the motor terminal from effective contact with the skeletal muscle fibre (Vrbová and Lowrie, 1989).

7.5   ... Abnormal changes in their state or environment

The subtitle of this section is taken from the definition of plasticity given by Brown and Hardman (1987). The definition has been used previously in this book. There will be no talk of *atrophy* of disuse or of *hypertrophy* following exercise. That would presume an understanding of *trophic* actions as nerve influences skeletal muscle. It would need an understanding also of the difficult concept of *neurotrophicity* which will be introduced below.

Physical activity increases in a person the ability to perform physical work; a period of physical inactivity decreases it. Looking more closely at those statements we must discuss them in terms which are relevant to rehabilitation. Physical performance needs qualification by adding the ability to perform physical work *at specific rates and for specific durations of time*. The major points of this approach to neuromuscular plasticity and rehabilitation have been drawn in part from Saltin (1985).

It should be realized that outside the laboratory, and in the realm of the whole human, it is a system that is adapting, and not simply a tissue. This returns us of course to FORMFUNCTION which cannot be better illustrated than by discussing the participation of the molecular components of skeletal muscle and also of the cardiovascular and respiratory systems as components of total plastic adaptation of the neuromuscular elements of the skeletomotor system.

An increasing physical activity can take the form of a therapy which includes a planned component of physical conditioning. This brings about an increase in the capillary density of postural muscles as well as a concomitant adaptation of the enzymes of skeletal muscle. This adaptation of enzyme activity will determine the preferential paths of the metabolism the muscle will follow as a consequence. An experimental approach to this adaptation is given by Hudlická *et al.* (1977). Briefly, electrical stimulation in a steady pattern delivered at a mean frequency of 10 stimuli per second was applied in experimental animals. It induced the transformation from anaerobic to aerobic metabolism. This was deduced from an increase in capillary density (the number of blood capillaries per skeletal muscle fibre), from an increase in oxidative metabolism of the skeletal muscle and from an increase in the activity of the enzyme ATPase in the sarcoplasmic reticulum of the skeletal muscle fibres. This example of system adaptation in plasticity of skeletal muscle, along with others, is discussed in particular by Vrbová *et al.* (1978) and, in relationship to human thigh muscle, by Saltin (1985).

It is appropriate at this stage of the book to introduce again a cautionary note about relating the patterns of stimulation employed during an electrotherapy to what you know now about molecular neurobiology. The starting point will be the regulation of free Ca^{2+} in the sarcoplasm of a muscle fibre and the action of that ion on the ATPase of skeletal muscle (see Chapter 1, page 9). *The enzyme ATPase transfers the 'high energy' of the two terminal phosphate bonds of ATP to energetic processes of the skeletal muscle fibre. Two of these processes are important to the caution being suggested. The first is the role of the free Ca^{2+} on myofibrillar ATPase.* The myosin molecules have a 'head' and a 'tail' or, to be more precise, a heavy and a light meromyosin. The ATP binds to a binding site on the heads of heavy meromyosin throughout the myofibril (Fig. 7.5). Free Ca^{2+} is released from its place of sequestration in the sarcoplasmic reticulum by the invasion of action currents generated by each nerve impulse or every electrical stimulus. The starting place for a discussion of free Ca^{2+} is the natural or the electrotherapeutically induced action potential (See Fig. 7.5a). This is propagated from the motor point of the muscle fibres over the muscle fibre membranes. The surface over which the potential is propagated (smoothly and not by saltation) includes the (transverse) T-canals which run at right angles to the long axis of the fibres. There is one of these trans-

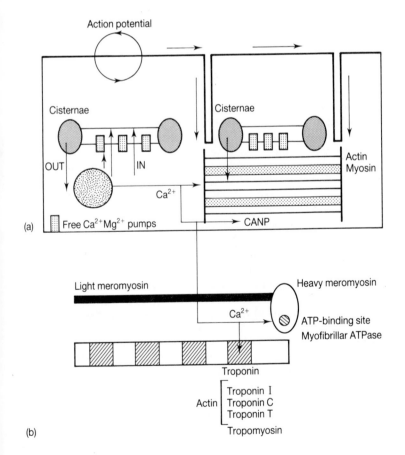

Fig. 7.5 The action of free Ca^{2+} released from its site of sequestration in the sites of the sarcoplasmic reticulum (dumbell-shaped) structures of adjacent sarcomeres in a myofibril. (a) The effect of action potentials in the T-system running into the depth of the myofibril is to release freed Ca^{2+} into the sarcoplasm. It remains there as free ion until the action potential has ended. It is then pumped, to be sequestered in the reticulum by the action of Mg^{2+} pumps. If a muscle is excited more frequently than the rate at which sequestration can occur, the free Ca^{2+} is able to extend its range of action to CANP (see text). (b) The sites of free Ca^{2+} action on the process of excitation/mechanical action coupling.

verse canal systems at the border of the sarcomere. The action potential, or the effect of the current generated by it, is transferred to the membrane of the cisternae of the sarcoplasmic reticulum. This releases Ca^{2+} from the reservoir in the sarcoplasmic reticulum where it has been held by the protein calsequestrin (see Fig. 7.6). The free Ca^{2+} at this stage of mechanical action of the muscle fibres has two modes of action. The first is to engage as intermediary one of the complex of four molecules associated with actin (see Fig. 7.5b). In this position, the Ca^{2+} is able to activate the myofibrillar ATPase and place the heavy meromyosin into an active form whereupon it performs the 'rowing action' of the actin/myosin molecules. The heavy meromyosin switches to an inactivated 'reverse stroke' in the rowing, ready for and in response to the next action potential, to resume its active state and take another pull on the oar of muscular action.

In the second mode of action, the free Ca^{2+} is able to activate the neutral protease (see CANP in Chapter 1, p. 9). The time of transition in the states of Ca^{2+} from sequestered to free and back again to sequestered is critical in a response to an electrotherapy. Should there be a mismatch between the frequency of electrical stimulation and the timing of the cycles of states of the Ca^{2+} the rehabilitative purpose of the electrotherapy could be opposed by a stimulation-induced proteolysis. The muscle fibres could then be transformed into a form of nutrient broth and not into muscle fibres adapted by plastic adaptation to be more effective

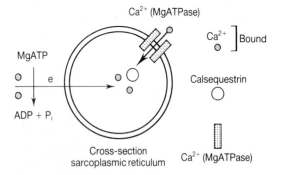

Fig. 7.6 A diagram illustrating the role of calsequestrin in determining the ratio of time during which the Ca^{2+} occupies the 'bound' and 'free' forms in the sarcoplasm. This determines in which phase the ion is going to act. Also shown is the molecular complex which regulates the ionic forms of Ca^{2+}: the Ca^{2+}, MgATPase is an enzyme which is activated by Ca^{2+} and then releases the bond energy of ATP and applies it to an ion pump, specific for the Ca^{2+}.

in movement. Protein synthesis required for an effective rehabilitation could utilize the digestion products providing that the pattern of the electrotherapy permits it so to do, or better still carries a 'trophic code' which encourages it to do so.

7.6   Activity-induced plastic adaptation of skeletal muscle

Pette and Vrbová (1985) argue cogently that activity is a major factor in determining the phenotype of skeletal muscle. Activity should include as its components: inactivity, changes in activity, unnatural activity, disordered activity and induced activity. The ability to change the characteristics of skeletal muscle by modifying its role in these components of activity may give a measure of the mutability of muscle or even better, a measure of the responsiveness of muscle to changing activity. This particular point has been recognized previously. Edgerton *et al.* (1985) have asked 'what is the flexibility of the neural control of muscle properties?' An answer to that question can be found only if we explore the patterns of activity to which a skeletal muscle is subjected.

One of the key laboratory observations is that several months after cross re-uniting their nerves, cut experimentally (Buller *et al.* 1960; Close, 1969), a slow-twitch muscle can be converted towards a fast-twitch muscle and vice versa. This is shown by appropriate changes in their times to contract, the times they take to relax to one-half of their peak contractile force (half relaxation time) and in their maximum velocities of shortening. It should be pointed out that once again these observations tell us more about the readiness with which the muscles respond by changing, rather than the true appropriateness of the procedure by which the changes are obtained.

Amongst the components of activity to which muscle shows plastic adaptation, induced activity is included. Electrical stimulation of the motor point of a muscle (the anatomical point within a muscle where motor axons innervate motor endplates) when it is carried out therapeutically, i.e. as an electrotherapy, comes under that category. Historically, electrotherapy has diverse forms. Faradism, interrupted Galvanism and interferential waveform stimulation are amongst them. There is no doubt that all forms have some effectiveness, but one has to ask again whether we are demonstrating the 'susceptibility' of muscle to adapt to various forms of induced activity rather than a special manner or pattern in which the activity is induced.

Although skeletal muscle is not a proficient linguist, it could be true to say that it undergoes a form of plastic adaptation 'when you speak to a muscle in a language it understands'. So it is really left to us to watch our words, or at least, our stimuli. It appears as though the pattern in which a train of electrical stimuli is given to a muscle (as electrotherapy, for example) is of some importance; more importantly still, a second meaning of stimulation is superimposed onto the first (Dayhoff and Gerstein, 1983a). This would appear to add semantics to the language instructing a plastic adaptation of the system to which the muscle belongs.

A pattern employed in electrical stimulation of a muscle is difficult to define. It could mean a pattern in time of electrical events when a waveform exceeds the threshold of the tissue for stimulation. The fact that a sinusoidal waveform is employed does not mean that the current flowing, with an amplitude as a continuum of time, and intended to be a stimulus is indeed a stimulus. Rectification by the tissue and the presence of a threshold to electrical stimulation punctuates the smooth waveform by introducing a pattern of threshold interspersed with subthreshold episodes of an applied stimulating current.

A pattern is better defined by Edgerton *et al.* (1985) when they distinguish between the controls that the motor nervous system has over the physiological and biochemical properties of skeletal muscle. Two of the neural controls they describe are: (1) the *quantity* of nerve impulses employed by the motoneurons, and (2) the *quality* of impulses the motoneurons supply to the responding muscle units (the *motor* unit comprises the motoneuron, its axon and branches, and all of the muscle fibres innervated by them. A *muscle* unit, by comparison, takes into account the muscle fibres only: the motoneuron and any influences upon it are not considered). In other words, the quality of impulses is both the number of impulses discharged and the pattern in which they are discharged.

Translating, with the purpose of describing electrotherapies, for *nerve impulses* you should read *threshold stimuli*. When a procedure of electrical stimulation is used as a therapy we must remember the definition of a stimulus as: '. . . any change in the environment which produces a response in an excitable tissue' (Benton *et al.*, 1981). That defi-

nition, which complements the one used by Brown and Hardman (1987), and has been used repeatedly in this book.

Something has to be added to the preceding definitions of stimulus. That is, a stimulus is an effective change in environment which enables us to distinguish between: (1) the component of the stimulus which has an immediate effect (the stimulus/response effect), and (b) the component of a stimulus which encourages an eventual adaptive plastic change in the system.

A stimulus has to be considered, therefore, as a dual event: (1) anything which produces a response in an excitable tissue, and (2) when it is applied for an appropriate length of time, anything which assumes the nature of a stressor (see Chapter 1) which will modify unavoidably any response by the tissue to further stimulation.

Such an hypothetical division of an episode of stimulation introduces a possibility that stimulation intended to be functional, in the conventional sense of bioENGINEERING, might not be what is intended. It could well be counter to what is intended if that is to fit the metabolic and mechanical properties of motor units to a desired motor effectiveness (Buchegger *et al.*, 1984; Goldspink, 1985).

An intentional transformation of a fast-twitch skeletal muscle, *tibialis anterior* (TA), into a slow-twitch muscle, resembling *extensor digitorum longus* (EDL) in motor action, was brought about by long-term electrical stimulation through electrodes implanted in experimental animals (Salmons and Vrbová, 1969). The uniform pattern of stimulation employed had a mean frequency of 10 Hz and so approximated closely the natural frequency at which EDL normally receives action potentials from its motoneuron pool. Similar observations on muscle transformation in laboratory animals have been made by Sarazalam *et al.* (1982) and Buchegger *et al.* (1984). Human electrotherapy was studied with great care by Scott *et al.* (1985). Hudlická *et al.* (1980) and Hudlická (1985) extended their animal studies to consider the microvasculature of skeletal muscle, and also the changing metabolic characteristics and mechanical performance of fast-twitch skeletal muscle.

We could say, yet again, that the techniques just described yield more knowledge of the readiness of skeletal muscle to undergo plastic adaptation than of the specificity of the patterns of stimulation used to bring the adaptation about. The use of different patterns of stimulation in electrotherapies reveals a great deal about the factors which best induce purposeful plastic adaptation of skeletal muscles. This they do by showing that the duration of their application is approximately related to the durations of episodes of normal motor behaviour.

A return to the importance of motor activity as a control factor in the induction and development of a purposeful plastic adaptation was made by Gibson *et al.* (1988). In a number of patients atrophy of the quadriceps developed in consequence of leg immobilization. This could be prevented if the muscle was stimulated electrically by a pattern of stimulation delivered percutaneously at 30 Hz. The pattern of stimulation was simple: repeated 2.0 s on/9.0 s off cycles were employed.

In a convincing way, Harris *et al.* (1982) demonstrated in rabbits stimulated with intermittent bursts of electric stimuli (40–60 Hz) that fast-twitch to slow-twitch transformation occurred as TA took on the characteristics of EDL. This was an observation similar to those seen in these muscles after prolonged low-frequency (10 Hz) electrical stimulation. Remarking pertinently Harris *et al.* (1982) report that the transformation is elicited by an increase in the *total amount* of contractile activity that is involved rather than the *frequency of* stimulation at which the contractile activity is developed.

7.7   . . . The silences between them

In a discussion of the beauty of the music of Mozart, it is sometimes said that beauty is not so much about the notes, but about the silences between them. It has been known for 60 years that the control of physiological systems is understood in terms of homeostasis: the maintenance of constancy of the internal environment of the body. Since 1969 there has been an alternative philosophy available.

Iberall (1969) suggested that the concept of homeostasis is too limiting to explain the subtleties of biocontrol. Contributing to the symposium 'Towards a Theoretical Biology' (Waddington, 1969), Iberall proposes two alternatives, either homeorrhoesis or homeokinesis. These mean, respectively, a stability of flow of both material and information, and a dynamic stability of systems in movement. One of the first benefits of this different approach to systems of control was developed by Kitney and Rompelman (1980) in their study of the variability of heart rate.

In brief, this theoretical analysis of the heart rate in humans asks us to accept that in an electrocardiogram there is as much, if not more, clinical information available in the intervals between successive points of the R–R peaks than there is in the PQRST waveforms which separate them. A general development of the information content of the electrocardiogram is offered by Saul (1990) in which he illustrates the power of this technique applied to an understanding of the roles in cardiac control systems of a modulation of cardiac autonomic outflow.

Discussing the frequency at which the several cardiac control systems operate, Saul emphasizes that they fall into three bands within the range 0.03 and 0.15 Hz. Attention is drawn also to the fact that the final common pathways for this control system are the vagal and sympathetic efferents. Dare we now translate R–R intervals in an electrocardiogram as intervals between action potential in trains of motoneuron discharge?

There are respectable precedents for this. The expression of a non-uniform frequency of discharge of action potentials by the unit Hertz (Hz) is incorrect (Lynn, 1987). A non-uniformity in the pattern of discharge recorded from motoneurons and motor units has been reported (Baldissera and Kernell, 1984; Kernell, 1984). Those workers give a clear indication that expression of frequency must not assume its uniformity, because that accepts automatically the calculation of a mean. Instead, the mean must be expanded first by taking into consideration the variance of the mean, and from that to more refined analyses.

A static analysis which involves mean frequency and the deviation from that mean, taken together with an analysis involving the distribution frequency (in the mathematical sense) is little better than a snap-shot when what is required is a video-film of the pattern of motoneuron discharge from which a model of electrotherapy pattern can be obtained. This pattern of discharge of a motoneuron or motor unit discharge is correctly referred to as a point process, or more generally a stochastic point process (Lynn, 1987). The mathematical power of such an analysis is seen clearly in the work of Clamann (1969) who has published a statistical analysis of motor unit firing patterns in human skeletal muscle. The dynamic mathematics required for this analysis is developed fully by Cox and Isham (1980).

A most significant early approach to the subject

of patterned neuron discharge, within the context of the present book, was made by Stein (1969). The examples of a re-introduction of patterns of stimulation derived from information carrying neurons in neural systems is interesting. Perkel, Gerstein and Moore (1969a and b) approach the likelihood of information being carried in the trains of action potentials of neurons in both of the cases of: (a) single spike trains and of (b) simultaneously discharging spike trains.

Dayhoff and Gerstein (1983a) divide a train of action potential transmitted by a single axon into two parts: a background train concerned with ongoing controls of the nervous system as it is found, and a 'favored pattern' which appears repeatedly and is concerned with information required to direct the plastic adaptation for a future function of the nervous system involved. An example of action potential trains analysed by Dayhoff and Gerstein was recorded from the striate cortex of the cat.

7.8 Trophicity and muscle transformation

Something of a digression at this point must be allowed into the run of the argument. Mention has been made already about atrophy, hypertrophy and trophicity (cf. Chapter 1, Section 1.2). The word 'trophic' derives from the Greek *trophe* (nourishment) and it became respectable in the discussion of the parameters of control and development in the widest aspect of biology. Trophism was used in discussions, for example, of the availability of nutrients, and then during the description of the utilization of food chains in the biological kingdom. The word was brought into use specifically with respect to the long-term influences of nerve upon nerve, and of nerve upon skeletal muscle. An example of exact usage is by Vrbová (1989) who, in a discussion of the multiple controlling influence that nerve has upon muscle, describes '(1) mechanisms that operate during conduction and synaptic (endplate) transmission triggering muscle contraction, a mechanism that operates, for example, in the trophic effect of training; (2) specific neurotrophic influences independent of nerve impulses'. This quotation reveals the foresight of Gutmann (1969) when he wrote 'When considering the maintenance influence of muscle mediated by the nerve a multiple control of maintenance must be assumed'.

Candidates proposed as neurotrophic agents in the maintenance are: (1) acetylcholine released in connection with the production of miniature endplate potentials (MEPPs) (Fatt and Katts, 1952; Thesleff, 1960; Drachman, 1967); (2) the transsynaptic transfer of chemical agents other than acetylcholine; and (3) mechanisms acting in addition to humoral regulation. These could include energy substrates and hormones carried in lymph formed by transcapillary transfer.

We should mention here that Gutmann (1969) described a denervation as 'atrophy which takes longer to develop when the length of the remaining peripheral stump of the sectioned nerve is also long'. The converse is true additionally when the nerve is cut close to the muscle. The conduction of nerve impulses ceases simultaneously in both cases of nerve transection. Approximately, for example, for each additional cm in length of the remaining nerve stump, endplate degeneration in rat diaphragm is delayed by 45 min. A reservoir of axoplasm retaining as yet unidentified trophic substances *en route* for terminal structures seems likely.

Price (1974) extends the concept of neurotrophism in his discussion of the influence the periphery has on the activity of spinal motoneurons. It is possible to think of the existence of a 'trophic loop' whereby a feedback loop exists between centre and periphery. We can extend this concept to include possibly an interaction of a nerve centre, operating in feedback, upon another nerve centre. Figure 7.7 illustrates this operation.

7.9 Guiding neuromuscular plasticity by eutrophic electrotherapy

An advance from electrotherapies based on a mean frequency, i.e. a uniform pattern of discharge, was attempted by Kidd and Oldham (1988a). With this technique, a full interference pattern of motor unit action potentials (MUAPs) was recorded from *first dorsal interosseus* of a normal hand during the application of maximum voluntary force with the finger operating in abduction and in an isometric state.

An analysing technique resolved the complexity of the EMG signal (Kidd and Oldham, 1988a) using an analytical electromyographic procedure. This allowed extraction of a sequence of interspike intervals from a single MUAP which was identified as being fatigue resistant. The MUAP firing pattern was far from uniform but had a mean fre-

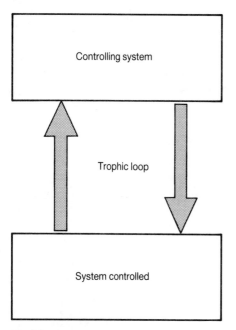

Fig. 7.7 A trophic loop can form at all levels of the CNS. We have discussed at length the molecular events involved in plastic adaptation. We must now face the possibility that one adapted centre or level in the CNS can impress the change it has shown itself on another centre or level in the CNS. A controlling system can modify by adaptation a system it controls. The cycle can be repeated until you are satisfied by the neuromuscular plastic adaptation you have achieved.

quency of firing of 9.8 Hz. The same motor unit was sampled when it was in an unfatigued state. It was also sampled after it had been fatigued by repeated maximal isometric action to the point where it could generate a force of only 65% of maximum voluntary force (MVF) and it was sampled finally after isometric action to a point where it could generate only 30% of maximum MVF. The second series of analyses had once again a mean frequency of discharge of approximately 10 Hz. The full pattern of the three discharges, when considered as point processes, were strikingly different. The three patterns were 'programmed' into a CMOS microchip which was used to control a personal stimulator. The patterns of MUAP discharge were replicated exactly in this way.

A clinical trial of this eutrophic electrotherapy was carried out with patients whose *first dorsal interossei* had atrophied as a consequence of the pain and the disuse of the arthritic hand. Neither physiotherapy nor any administration of drugs had preceded or accompanied the trial of the electro-

therapy. In essence, a natural discharge pattern detected from a normal hand and recorded into a stimulator was replayed as an electrotherapy into the atrophied muscles of arthritic patients.

A clinical trial was carried out to test the effectiveness of eutrophic electrotherapy by comparing its effect with that of electrotherapy applying a uniform pattern of stimulation to the muscle with a mean frequency of approximately 10 Hz. In an additional element of the trial, stimulation containing a random reordering of the MUAP pattern was incorporated. It has been pointed out (Lynn, 1987) that there is a paucity of information present, in the sense of an ability to direct plastic adaptation of a muscle, if a signal carried by a train of stimuli is presented in a uniform pattern: i.e. one that has been simplified to a mean frequency. As Lynn states, no additional information is transmitted by the train of stimuli after the first interstimulus interval has been passed.

The MUAP pattern was taken from a normal muscle after it had been fatigued to a state where it could not deliver more than 30% of its original, unfatigued voluntary force. The effect of that electrotherapy was compared with that of a uniform pattern at 10 Hz. The uniform pattern had some slight effect and the randomly reordered signal had no effect at all. The simplest analysis of the results is presented as in Figs 7.8a, b and 7.9a, b. Note that the endurance measured in Figs 7.8a and b are over different scales.

Figures 7.9a and b again compare the effectiveness of the two different electrotherapies. This time the measure used was the MVF attainable by the patients. The difference in effectiveness of the two electrotherapies lead us to call the natural pattern *eutrophic*, by which name we mean one that has been calculated as being ideal in initiating a purposeful plastic adaptation by the muscle to be treated. The comparison of the two different forms of electrotherapy was made by measuring (1) the effectiveness in bringing about a change in endurance of the muscle, and (2) the maximal isometric force which could be developed by it. The therapy was administered for three hours each day for 10 weeks. Full details of the procedure will be found in Kidd *et al.* (1989).

The results are expressed as the percentage change in the parameter measured from a control value obtained from a patient who performed the full range of appropriate testing procedure *but received no electrotherapy of whatever form.* All of the

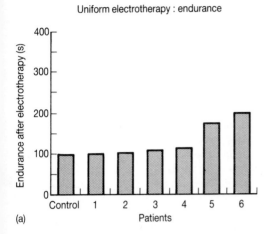

(a)

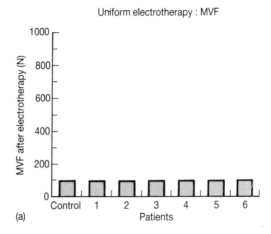

(a)

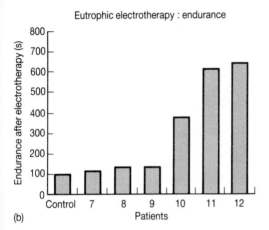

(b)

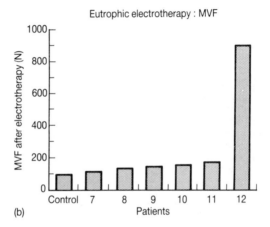

(b)

Fig. 7.8 (a) The endurance with which maximum voluntary force (MVF) could be held until it dropped to 50% of its initial value. The figure shows the results of six patients receiving uniform electrotherapy and the improvement in endurance after 10 weeks of electrotherapy given three hours each day. The results from the patients are ranked in order of effectiveness. Note that the time scales for endurance after the two electrotherapies are different. (b) Six different patients received an identical duration of electrotherapy as those in Fig. 7.8a, but in this case the pattern was eutrophic. Note again that the time scales for endurance after the two electrotherapies are different.

Fig. 7.9 (a) A repeat of the comparison of the effectiveness of patterns of electrotherapy. Here, a uniform pattern had either no effect, or a deleterious effect on maximum voluntary force (MFV) which could be developed before and after electrotherapy. Further details are in the text. (b) By comparison, a eutrophic pattern was effective in improving force generation in all patients and remarkably so in one of them (no. 12).

control values have been called 100%. The control measurement was taken from patients who followed the full and appropriate testing procedure in case it possibly gave some training effect on its own. These values are shown as the first, left-hand column of each graph. The results obtained with the patients who participated in the trial are ranked according to the effectiveness of the respective

electrotherapy. With this form of analysis, the electrotherapy, expressed as a uniform pattern reproducing only a mean frequency, is less effective than the eutrophic pattern in that it confers a smaller increase in endurance on the muscles, and it shows signs of being countereffective in developing an increase in isometric force.

A more detailed analysis (Figs 7.10a, b) offers values calculated from the average response from all six patients participating in each part of the trial. A simple regression analysis has been per-

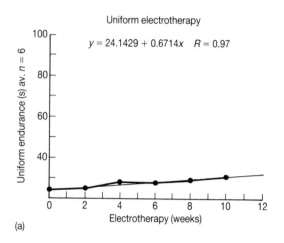

Uniform electrotherapy

$y = 24.1429 + 0.6714x$ $R = 0.97$

(a)

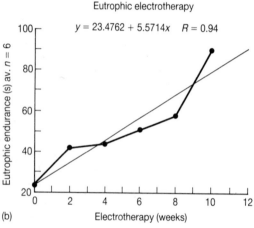

Eutrophic electrotherapy

$y = 23.4762 + 5.5714x$ $R = 0.94$

(b)

Fig. 7.10   (a) The average ability of six patients to endure maximum voluntary force (MVF) development during 10 weeks of electrotherapy of uniform frequency. All patients showed an improvement in endurance. (b) By comparison, eutrophic electrotherapy gave great improvement in the average endurance of all six patients.

formed for each set of results. The slope of the line *x* shows whether the endurance or force developed by the hand in some parts of the trial is increasing (whereupon *x* adopts a positive value) or is decreasing (*x* adopts a negative value). The value *R* is an indicator of the reliability of the average value which contributed to the regression. Numerically, a value for *R* between 0 and 1 is possible. When *R* = 1 it means that all of the variability in effectiveness of the electrotherapies is explained. All of the values of *R* obtained in this trial are acceptable as a basis for the argument which follows.

Two features of the six-patient trial will be used to support the argument. The effectiveness of a uni-

form electrotherapy with a mean frequency of 10 Hz is compared to an eutrophic pattern. The results are illustrated in Figs 7.10a and b, in which the procedures tested were the ability to develop maximal voluntary, isometric force and the endurance with which that force could be applied until it had dropped to 50% of that maximum. The uniform electrotherapy decreased the development of maximal force in two of the six patients, and gave an increase in the four remaining patients which was not accessible to statistical procedures with the form of analysis used.

By comparison, episodes of eutrophic electrotherapy developed, in those patients who received it, a remarkable increase in both endurance and maximal voluntary development of isometric force. Decreases in maximal isometric force development has been described previously with uniform pattern electrotherapy and a mixed frequency electrotherapy was adopted by some workers in an attempt to spare the muscle from this reduction of force development.

The more refined statistical analysis in Figs 7.11a and b allows a more telling presentation of the results from the clinical trial. Note how the effects of eutrophic electrotherapy by comparison with the effects of the uniform pattern electrotherapy gave rise to an increased slope of the line describing the change in hand grip obtained. Note also how the eutrophic electrotherapy reversed the slope of the line describing the increase in development of maximal force on voluntary action. Additionally, the eutrophic electrotherapy increased the steepness of the slope at which the force of hand grip increased during the 10 weeks of electrotherapy.

When the results from these trials have been confirmed by an independent laboratory this start in the search for a more meaningful pattern of electrotherapy will have been justified. The small sample of 6.5 s of MUAP discharge pattern from a normal muscle in a state of near fatigue and replicated as an electrotherapy, where it is repeated time and time again, for three hours each day over 10 weeks, seems able to confer the state of plastic adaptation in a skeletal muscle which counteracts the tendency towards weakness and fatiguability.

The time for which the interspike intervals of a single motor unit have been measured has been increased, again in the laboratory, to 25 s and this pattern has been shown to have further advantages as an electrotherapy (Dale, 1990, personal com-

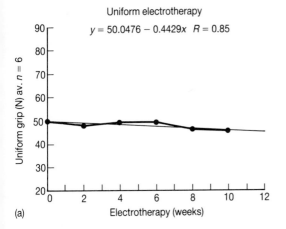

Uniform electrotherapy

$$y = 50.0476 - 0.4429x \quad R = 0.85$$

(a)

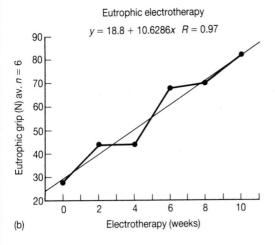

Eutrophic electrotherapy

$$y = 18.8 + 10.6286x \quad R = 0.97$$

(b)

Fig. 7.11   (a) The average force developed by six patients who received an electrotherapy of uniform pattern for 10 weeks. All six patients showed a reduction in their ability to generate force (the value of *x* took on a negative value) with full hand grip as the therapy progressed. (b) A different six patients from those illustrated in Fig. 7.10a responded to eutrophic electrotherapy applied for 10 weeks by showing a greatly improved ability (the value of *x* in the relative equation takes a positive value) to generate force by full hand grip. The point of application of the therapy was localized to the motor point of the first dorsal interosseus. A discussion of the possible mechanism of this improvement in full hand grip is introduced in the text.

munication). An earlier electrotherapy utilizing a mean frequency pattern of discharge from active and normal facial muscles of expression in humans has proved in clinical trial to be effective in its own right, and to act as an adjuvant to conventional physiotherapy (Farragher *et al.*, 1987).

7.10   Are you sure about exactly which structures you are stimulating?

You may have your stimulating electrode applied to the skin surface over the motor point of a super-ficial muscle, but that does not mean that you are stimulating only those motor axons that are *en route* to the muscle. You should realize that what you are stimulating are all those excitable tissues whose electrical threshold is below or falls below the charge transfer of the stimuli. The potency of natu-ral motoneuron signals, replicated as electrother-apy stimuli must not be underestimated. Some of the neuromuscular elements understanding the language transmitted by the signal are illustrated by Fig. 7.12. In addition to the orthodromic stimu-lation of the intended axons, antidromic stimu-lation of the same axons, which was probably not intended, is also brought about.

The antidromic potentials in response to each stimulus invade the soma of the motoneuron by way of the initial segment of the axon and the axon hillock from which it extends. As the pathway by which an action potential generated naturally invades the soma and possibly the dendrites is simi-lar to the one followed by artificially generated potentials we should expect the motoneuron not to be able to distinguish the two. The therapeutic effect of this similarity in movement rehabilitation cannot be underestimated.

Why, for example, does a rehabilitation of a full hand movement, such as grip, follow eutrophic electrotherapy applied in a localized manner to the motor point of first dorsal interosseus (Fig. 7.9b)?

Could it be, possibly, that a microiontophoresis by the action currents invading the soma membrane moves the macromolecules in the motoneuron membrane (Poo, 1985)? This action could well be a part of the full plastic adaptation of the *motor* unit and not a simple transformation of the *muscle* unit only. Furthermore, the antidromic invasion of recurrent collaterals of the motor axons involve the Renshaw system in the full adaptive response. We should not forget that afferent axons of appropriate electrical threshold will be involved also in the response to a stimulation train. The orthodromic action of these could well condition the activity of synapses on the motoneurons and their interneu-rons. We feel that this general phase of involvement contributes significantly to the great differences between an electrotherapy which brings about a simple modification of skeletal muscle fibre charac-

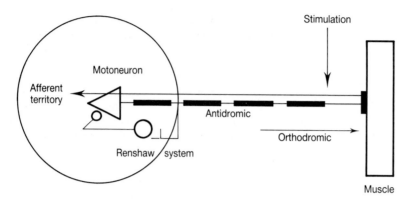

Fig. 7.12 At times, too little thought is given to the systems affected by localized electrotherapy. Stimuli localized to the motor point of a muscle can stimulate axons other than the ones intended. This diagram illustrates the bombardment of the motoneuron pool by the consequences of the stimulation. Further discussion is presented in the text.

teristics, and one which gives full movement rehabilitation.

7.11   Look to the future with vigour and not with a fondness on the past

This chapter has introduced you to some of the macromolecules which are at the heart of plastic adaptation in skeletal muscle. Some of the fundamental features of its embryology have been introduced. How there can be also a recapitulation of certain stages of embryological development is discussed. Electrical stimulation of nerve and muscle in the past has involved a stimulus/response approach. The electrotherapy has supplied only the 'background train' of Dayhoff and Gerstein (1983a) which produces an immediate response and muscle twitching. There could be a warning here about using, unthinkingly, the range of frequencies available on some electrotherapy instruments. Remember that the characteristics of skeletal muscle have been formed by contact with a motoneuron on the motor unit. They have also responded to the discharge pattern of action potentials delivered to them by the motoneuron. There is, for that reason, a naturally maintained match of motoneuron activity and the characteristics of the muscle fibres it innervates. Any mismatch between these characteristics could disturb possibly the molecular balance of the muscle fibres. The effect of CANPs, as discussed in Chapter 1 with respect to the autoproteolysis of muscle substance, must be recognized now. A close match of muscle fibres and the pattern of discharge of their motoneurons must be obtained. It is for that reason that the eutrophic pattern introduced into electrotherapies (see above) has been studied. There is the awful possi-

bility that a frequency of stimulation applied to a muscle higher than the mean firing frequency of firing of its motoneurons could turn the sarcoplasm into a form of nutrient broth rather than develop the desired plastic adaptation of the skeletal muscle. The search into the language of skeletal muscle has attempted to add the 'favoured pattern' which directs plastic adaptation and therefore improves muscle performance for the future. It is now up to those linguists in the professions of rehabilitation to weave more compelling statements from the loom of this language (Affeldt, 1988) and persuade the processes of plastic adaptation to meet better their professional requirements.

References

Affeldt, J. E. (1988) The tapestry of rehabilitation, its weavers and its threads. *Journal of Allied Health* **2**: 53–8.

Baldissera, F. and Kernell, D. (1984) Impulse frequency coding of the dynamic effects of excitation. *Archives Italienes de Biologie* **122**: 43–58.

Benton, L. A., Baker, L. L., Bowman, B. R. and Waters, R. L. (1981) *Functional Electrical Stimulation – A Practical Clinical Guide*. Downey, California: Professional Staff Association, Rancho Los Amigos Hospital.

Brown, M. A. and Hardman, V. J. (1987) Plasticity of vertebrate motoneurons. In Winlow, W. and McCrohan, C. eds. *Growth and Plasticity of Neural Connections*. Manchester: Manchester University Press, pp. 36–51.

Buchegger, A., Nemeth, P. M., Pette, D. and Reichmann, H. (1984) Effects of chronic stimulation of different patterns in the metabolic heterogeneity of the fibre population in rabbit tiabilis anterior muscle. *Journal of Physiology* **350**: 109–19.

Buller, A. J., Eccles, J. C. and Eccles, R. M. (1960) Differentiation of fast and slow muscles in the cat hind limb. *Journal of Physiology* **150**: 399–416.

Burke, R. E., Levine, N., Salcman, M. and Trairis, P. (1974) Motor units in cat soleus muscle: physiological, histochemical and morphological characteristics. *Journal of Physiology* **238**: 503–14.

Clamann, H. P. (1969) Statistical analysis of motor unit firing patterns in human skeletal muscle. *Biophysical Journal* **10**: 1233–51.

Close, R. (1969) Dynamic properties of fast and slow skeletal muscle of the rat after nerve cross-union. *Journal od Physiology* **294**: 331–46.

Cox, D. R. and Isham, V. (1980) *Point Processes*. London: Chapman and Hall.

Dayhoff, J. E. and Gerstein, G. L. (1983a) Favored patterns in spike trains. I. Detection. *Journal of Neurophysiology* **49**: 1334–48.

Dayhoff, J. E. and Gerstein, G. L. (1983b) Favored patterns in spike trains. II. Application. *Journal of Neurophysiology* **49**: 1349–63.

Drachmann, D. B. (1967) Is acetylcholine the trophic neuromuscular transmitter? *Archives of Neurology* **17**: 206–18.

Drachmann, D. B. (1974) Trophic functions of the neuron. *Annals of the New York Academy of Sciences* **228**.

Edgerton, V. R., Martin, T. P., Bodine, S. C. and Roy, R. R. (1985) How flexible is the neural control of muscle properties? *Journal of Experimental Biology* **115**: 393–402.

English, A. W. M. and Wolf, S. L. (1982) The motor unit: anatomy and physiology. *Phys. Therapy* **62**: 1763–85.

Faragher, D., Kidd, G. L. and Tallis, R. C. (1987) Eutrophic electrical stimulation for Bell's palsy. *Clinical Rehabilitation* **1**: 265–71.

Fatt, P. and Katz, B. (1952) Spontaneous subthreshold activity in motor nerve end-plates. *Journal of Physiology* **117**: 109–20.

Gibson, J. N. A., Rennie, M. J. and Smith, K. (1988) Prevention of disuse atrophy by means of electrical stimulation: maintenance of protein synthesis. *Lancet* **ii**: 767–9.

Goldspink, G. (1985) Malleability of the motor system: a comparative approach. *Journal of Experimental Biology* **118**: 375–91.

Guba, F. (1980) Facts and thoughts on muscle-fibre types. *Advances in Physiological Science* **24**: 1–16.

Guba, F., Marechal, G. and Taka'cs, O. (1980) *The Mechanisms of Muscle Adaptation to Functional Requirements*. Oxford: Pergamon.

Gutmann, E. (1969) The trophic function of the nerve cell. *Scientia* **194**: 1–20.

Harris, B., Heilig, A., Hudlická, O., Leberer, E., Pette, D. and Tyler, K. (1982) Changes in rabbit muscle enzyme activities response to chronic stimulation with different frequency patterns. In Pernow, X. and Saltin, B., eds. *Metabolic and Functional Changes During Exercise*.

Hudlická, O. (1985) Development and adaptability of microvasculature in skeletal muscle. *Journal of Experimental Biology* **115**: 215–28.

Hudlická, O., Brown, M. D., Cotter, M., Smith, M. and Vrbová, G. (1977) The effect of long term stimulation of fast muscles on their blood flow, metabolism and ability to stand fatigue. *Pflug. Arch. ges. Physiol.* **369**: 141–9.

Hudlická, O., Tyler, K. R. and Altman, T. (1980) The effect of long-term stimulation on fuel uptake and performance in fast skeletal muscle. In Pette, D. ed. *Plasticity of Muscle*. Berlin: de Guyter.

Iberall, A. S. (1969) New thoughts on bio-control. In Waddington, C. H. ed. *Towards a Theoretical Biology. 2. Sketches*. IUBS Symposium. Edinburgh: Edinburgh University Press.

Kernell, D. (1984) The meaning of discharge rate: excitation-to-frequency transduction as studied in spinal motoneurons. *Archivs Italia de Biologia* **122**: 5–15.

Kidd, G. L. and Oldham, J. A. (1988a) Motor unit action potentials (MUAP) sequence and electrotherapy. *Clinical Rehabilitation* **2**: 23–33.

Kidd, G. L. and Oldham, J. A. (1988b) An electrotherapy based on the natural sequence of motor unit action potentials: a laboratory trial. *Clinical Rehabilitation* **2**: 125–38.

Kidd, G. L., Oldham, J. A. and Stanley, J. K. (1989) Eutrophic electrotherapy and atrophied muscles: a pilot clinical trial. *Clinical Rehabilitation* **2**: 219–30.

Kitney, R. I. and Rompleman, O. (1980) *The Study of Heart Rate Variability*. Oxford: Clarendon Press.

Kugelberg, E. and Edström, L. (1968) Differential histochemical effects of muscle contractions on phosphorylase and glycogen in various types fibres: relation to fatigue. *Journal of Neurology, Neurosurgery and Psychiatry* **31**: 415–23.

Lynn, P. A. (1987) *An Introduction to the Analysis and Processing of Signals*. London: Macmillan Education.

MacConnail, M. A. and Basmajian, J. V. (1969) *Muscles and Movement: A Basis for Human Kinesiology*. Baltimore: Williams & Wilkins.

Perkel, D. H., Gerstein, G. L. and Moore, G. P. (1969a) Neuronal spike trains and stochastic processes I. The single spike train. *Biophysical Journal* **7**: 391–418.

Perkel, D. H., Gerstein, G. L. and Moore, G. P. (1969b) Neuronal spike trains and stochastic processes II. Simultaneous spike trains. *Biophysical Journal* **7**: 419–40.

Pernow, B. and Saltin, B. (1986). In Saltin, B. International Series on Sports Sciences. **16**; Biochemistry of Exercise. Illinois: Champaign.

Pette, D. (1984) Activity-induced fast to slow transitions in mammalian muscle. *Medical Science in Sports and Exercise* **16**: 517–528.

Pette, D. (1985) Metabolic heterogeneity of muscle fibres. *Journal of Experimental Biology* **115**: 179–89.

Pette, D. and Vrbová, G. (1985) Neural control of phenotype expression in mammalian muscle fibres. *Muscle Nerve* **8**: 676–89.

Poo, M-M. (1985) Mobility and localization of proteins in excitable membranes. *Annual Review of Neuroscience* **8**: 369–406.

Price, D. L. (1974) The influence of the periphery on spinal motoneurons. In Drachman, D. B. *Annals of the New York Academy of Sciences* **228**: 235–48.

Salmons, S. and Henrikkson, J. (1981) The adaptive response of skeletal muscle to increased use. *Muscle Nerve* **4**: 94–106.

Salmons, S. and Vrbová, G. (1969) *J. Physiol. (Lond.)* **201**: 535–49.

Saltin, B. (1985) Malleability of the system in overcoming limitations: structural elements. *Journal of Experimental Biology* **115**: 345–54.

Sarazalam, M. G., Szymanska, G., Wiehrer, W. and Pette, D. (1982) Effects of chronic stimulation at low frequency on the lipid phases of sarcoplasmic reticulum in rabbit fast twitch muscle. *European Journal of Biochemistry* **123**: 241–5.

Saul, J. P. (1990) Beat-to-beat variations of heart rate reflect modulation of cardiac autonomic outflow. *News in Physiological Science* **5**: 32–7.

Scott, O. M., Vrbová, G., Hyde, S. A. and Dubowitz, V. (1985) Effects of chronic low frequency stimulation on normal human tibialis anterior muscle. *Journal of Neurology, Neurosurgery and Psychiatry* **44**: 774-81.

Sherrington (1904) The correlation of reflexes as the principle of the common final path. *British Association* **74**: 728–41.

Spielholtz, N. I. (1982) Skeletal muscle: a review of its development *in vivo* and *in vitro*. *Physical Therapy* **62**: 1765–87.

Stein, R. B. (1969) The information capacity of nerve cells using a frequency code. *Biophysical Journal* **7**: 797–826.

Thesleff, S. (1960) Effects of motor innervation on the chemical sensitivity of skeletal muscle. *Physiological Review* **40**: 734–52.

Tyldesley, B. and Grieve, J. I. (1989) *Muscles, Nerves and Movement. Kinesiology in Daily Living*. Oxford: Blackwell Scientific Publications.

Vrbová, G. (1989) The concept of neuromuscular plasticity. In Rose, F. C., Jones, R. and Vrbová, G. eds. *Neuromuscular Stimulation: Basic Concepts and Clinical Implications*. New York: Demos Publications.

Vrbová, G., Gordon, T. and Jones, R. (1978) *Nerve-Muscle Interaction*. London: Chapman and Hall.

Vrbová, G. and Lowrie, M. (1989) Role of activity in developing synapses: search for molecular mechanisms. *News in Physiological Science* **4**: 75–8.

Vrbová, G., Navarrette, R. and Lowrie, M. (1985) Matching of muscle properties and motoneurone firing patterns during early stages of development. *Journal of Experimental Biology* **115**: 113–23.

Waddington, C. H. (1960) *Towards a Theoretical Biology. 2. Sketches*. IUBS Symposium. Edinburgh: Edinburgh University Press.

Chapter 8

Mechanisms of plasticity in development and redevelopment

8.1 Formation of new connections
8.2 Increasing synaptic effectiveness

8.3 Concluding remarks

Adaptive neuronal plasticity is the result of one of two main processes: either the formation of new connections, or the enhanced effectiveness of existing connections. This chapter is an outline of the mechanisms which might be responsible. It should be appreciated that plasticity is the subject of very active research and our understanding is far from complete. The picture presented here is therefore intended as only one version of the story so far, not the final account, and readers should bear in mind that concepts can change very rapidly in an actively researched field.

Why, then, present an incomplete version? Why go into such fine molecular detail, apparently far removed from the practice of most therapies? The justification for giving so much cellular and molecular detail is that any therapeutic technique which works, works through these (or equivalent) mechanisms. The reason for giving an incomplete account, apparently prematurely, is that eventually there must be a two-way interaction between effective therapeutic practice and laboratory research, and only practical trial will sift out those theories which are clinically relevant. In short, attempts to exploit theories will help to refine them and might, in the best circumstances, even replace them with better theories. There is no reason why laboratory scientists should have all the fun. In this game, therapists can play too.

8.1 Formation of new connections

8.1.1 The growth cone

The key structure in the formation of new connections is an expanded region, known as the growth cone, found at the end of developing and redevelop-

ing nerve processes. Growth cones occur at the ends of both dendrites and axons, which are called neurites when the difference between them is not specified. Growth cones vary in diameter from 0.5 μm in unconducive environments to 1 μm in growth-promoting environments. From their free margins long, thin thread-like processes arise. These are called filopodia and although they are only 0.1–0.2 μm in diameter, they may be up to 50 μm long. Between the filopodia, thin veils of membrane, called lamellipodia, are draped. If the growth cone is likened to a hand, the filopodia are like fingers and the lamellipodia are the webs between the fingers.

To understand the mechanisms involved in growth, it is necessary to know something about the structure of neurites and growth cones. The neurite leading into the growth cone has a lipid cell membrane inside which is a cortex containing microfilaments in a criss-crossing lattice work running parallel to the cell membrane. Microfilaments are 6 nm in diameter (a nm is a thousandth of a μm, or a millionth of a mm). They are made of single molecules of actin, called monomers, joined together in a chain which is called a polymer. Inside the microfilamentous cortex there is a central core to the neurite, containing microtubules running parallel to the length of the neurite. Microtubules are much thicker than microfilaments, some 26 nm in diameter, and they are polymers of a protein called tubulin. Finally, alongside the microtubules there are neurofilaments which are about 10 nm in diameter. Attached to the central core of microtubules there are various organelles in the process of being transported along the axon. These organelles include vesicles, smooth endoplasmic reticulum (capable of storing and releasing calcium) and mitochondria (the respiratory factories of the cell). Microtubules form the railway tracks down which organelles are transported.

At the growth cone the microtubules penetrate into the thickened central region but the neurofilaments stop at the transition between neurite and cone. Organelles are transported along microtubules as far as the central region of the growth cone, but neither organelles nor microtubules usually penetrate to the peripheral fringe of the cone. The peripheral part of the cone is occupied by actin filaments, forming a lattice work under most of the membrane, but forming parallel arrays in filopodia and at points where the membrane is attached to the extracellular substrate. Myosin can be found at the roots of the filopodia. Sometimes rows of vesicles can be seen arranged along the length of the actin microfilaments. In places, these vesicles become attached to the cell membrane, fusing with it. There is also evidence of the reverse process, termed endocytosis, which is the pinching off of cell membrane to form coated vesicles which fuse with bags of degradative enzymes called lysosomes.

How does growth occur, and what chooses the direction of growth? To begin with, we will deal with the direction of growth, which is the responsibility of filopodia. The filopodia consist of a membrane made largely of fatty material, or lipid. There are several types of proteins embedded in the lipid membrane. These proteins form smaller particles than are found elsewhere in the cell membrane, and there are fewer of them. Among the particles there are ionophores, or ionic channels. Channels for sodium are rarer in the growth cone than elsewhere, but voltage-gated calcium channels are more common. This reflects the importance of the intracellular calcium concentration in elongation and directional changes of the neurite.

Some of these proteins are like immunoglobulins, the antibodies generally involved in the body's defence reactions. In filopodia, these antibody-like proteins are called integrins, and instead of binding to foreign antigens, they bind to components of the extracellular matrix. There are various large proteins in the extracellular matrix. Outside the central nervous system (CNS), the extracellular matrix proteins include collagen, fibronectin and laminin. There is no collagen within the CNS, but laminin is found on neuroepithelial cells in the early stages of development and it reappears during regenerative activity after injury. There are enough integrins in a growth cone to bind to about 1000 laminin molecules, but each filopodium probably binds to only one molecule of laminin.

Part of the integrin molecule lies outside the cell, where it binds to laminin. The second part of the integrin spans the lipid cell membrane. Finally, the third part lies within the filopodium, where it binds to another protein called talin. Talin, in its turn, is able to bind to actin. The story so far is that laminin forms a trail of adhesive clues along the path that the growth cone is intended to follow. A filopodium wanders by and if one of its integrin molecules happens to brush against an extracellular laminin molecule, the two stick together. This anchors the filopodium to the extracellular matrix. The internal part of the integrin molecule now changes shape so that, via talin, it binds to actin. Consequently the actin in the filopodium is aligned towards the cell membrane at those places where adhesion to extracellular laminin has taken place. Aligned microfilaments of actin interact with myosin at the root of the filopodium and tension is thereby generated.

The next step in the process is somewhat confused at present (Mitchinson and Kirschner, 1988). At one time it was thought that the actin–myosin contraction shortened the filopodium, heaving the cone towards the point of attachment, and dragging the neurite behind it. It is now clear, however, that the neurite grows partly like a railway track, new material being added at the growing end. Just as the rails, once laid, do not move, there is no actual forward movement of the neurite or its growth cone. In fact, visible components such as the actin microfilaments and particles in the cone membrane move backwards, towards the cell body. This is accompanied by forward movement of invisible components, the monomers from which the actin polymers are built. Just as in a railway, where unlaid rails are brought forwards to the end of the track and then laid, actin monomers are brought to the end of the filopodium. Once rails are laid, however, they become immobile. Unlike a railway, the polymerized microfilaments of actin move backwards, probably as a result of interaction with the myosin at the root of the filopodium. When monomer is laid down at a faster rate than the polymer moves backwards, the filopodium elongates; otherwise, the filopodium retracts. In general, filopodia are dynamic structures, perpetually growing longer or shorter, but rarely staying the same length.

Microtubules are polymers of tubulin. It was once thought that they were formed in the cell body and moved *en masse* towards the end of the neurite. Now it seems more likely that mature microtubules stay relatively still and new tubulin is transported down the axon to be added to the far end of each microtubule. Since most of the far ends are in the growth cone, most elongation of microtubules occurs there. By unknown mechanisms, the microtubules in the growth cone become orientated towards the parallel actin filaments in the filopodia. Perhaps the actin–myosin complex pulls formed microtubules towards itself, perhaps it encourages polymerization in its own direction, or perhaps microtubules grow randomly and only those pointing towards the actin–myosin complexes are stabilized, leaving the others to depolymerize. Whatever the mechanism, there is a preponderance of microtubules directed towards those parts of the cone where actin has been aligned by adhesion to the extracellular matrix.

As mentioned above, microtubules are the rails along which organelles are transported. When they are orientated towards the filopodia adhering to the extracellular matrix, the organelles travelling along them will be delivered to these points of attachment. Among the organelles so delivered are vesicles, inside-out bags of membrane. Prior to transportation, these vesicles are gathered in swellings of the neurite, called varicosities, some 20 μm proximal to the growth cone. After transportation, the newly arrived vesicles fuse with the cell surface and the vesicle membrane is added to the cell membrane. The newly inserted membrane contributes to the formation of lamellipodia, the veils draped between the filopodia. Approximately 60 vesicles provide sufficient membrane to create one lamellipodium. As more membrane is added, the web of lamellipodia moves nearer to the tips of the filopodia, making the latter appear to retract. From a distance, then, it looks as if the filopodia contract, pulling the growth cone forwards, whereas in fact lamellipodia are filling in the gap between adjacent filopodia, 'burying' them. The microfilamentous core of a filopodium is moving backwards as new monomers are added to the far end. The membrane on the outside is also moving backwards as new membrane is added distally and old membrane is endocytosed proximally. The forward movement of the cone is therefore actually an illusion.

Current beliefs are that although actin microfilaments generate tension, they are more to do with controlling the direction of growth than providing the motive force. Interference with actin polymerization by drugs such as cytochalasin does not prevent neurite growth, but does destroy its directionality. By contrast, microtubules are under compression, against which transportation can take place, and the motive force for elongation is derived from this.

The next step is for the inner regions of the lamellipodia, nearest the growth cone, to thicken. Organelles are brought inside the base of the lamellipodia, expanding them until they fill to the diameter of the growth cone. As the advancing lamellipodia thicken, the growth cone is undergoing a slimming process. Membrane is reabsorbed at its neck, where the cone joins the neurite. The organelles within the cone are transported forwards into the lamellipodia. The cone becomes thinner, decreasing in diameter until it is no thicker than the neurite. The actin microfilaments lose their parallel orientation towards the cell membrane and the adhesion to the extracellular matrix is broken. Neurofilaments from the neurite invade what was the cone, and the cone now becomes a part of the neurite. Meanwhile the lamellipodia have become the growth cone.

To summarize this complicated story: filopodia protrude from the growth cone in every direction at random. Usually they meet nothing of interest, in which case the rate at which the microfilamentous actin core is moved backwards by myosin exceeds the rate at which the new monomers are added to the far end, and the filopodia shorten again. Sometimes, however, an integrin receptor in the filopodium meets an extracellular matrix molecule such as laminin. Laminin and integrin adhere to each other, binding the filopodium to the extracellular matrix. The intracellular part of the integrin molecule is induced to bind, via talin, to actin. Actin filaments now align themselves in parallel towards the point of adhesion. In some way this influences microtubules to line themselves up towards the actin microfilaments, either because they are pulled upon by actin–myosin or because they grow randomly and actin–myosin stabilizes only the correctly orientated tubules. Either way, vesicles travel down the microtubules and are delivered to those points where the membrane is attached to the extracellular matrix. The vesicles are then inserted into the cell membrane, expanding it. The expanded regions form thin veils, lamellipodia, extending between the filopodia. As more membrane is added, the lamellipodia grow towards the filopodial tips. Meanwhile the bases of the lamellipodia thicken, fill with the organelles formerly confined to the central region of the growth cone, and eventually mature into new growth cone. The older part of the growth cone loses its organelles into the lamellipodia, and its membrane is taken up by endocytosis so that is slims down to the diameter of its neurite. Once neurofilaments invade it, the old cone is converted into a mature neurite. From the new cone, developed from lamellipodia, more filopodia extend, explore the extracellular matrix, then either retract or adhere to it. And so the restless cycle continues.

The direction of growth is therefore determined by chance encounters between integrin receptors on filopodia meeting laminin molecules in the extracellular matrix. If two filopodia pointing in different directions both encounter laminin molecules, the growth cone divides in two, and the neurite branches. Is is only at these branch points that neurites retain adhesion to the extracellular matrix. Laminin is expressed by neuroepithelial cells at exactly the time that new connections develop, and the integrin receptors to laminin are expressed in growing neurons simultaneously. Once connections have formed, neither laminin nor integrin are needed and the genes for both are switched off. Following injury, however, some signal switches the genes back on again and both proteins can be found in traumatized tracts. From the point of view of therapy, the crucial question to be answered is: 'What are the signals that switch laminin and integrin genes back on, and how may they be controlled so that expression occurs where and when it is wanted?'

8.1.2   Other adhesion molecules

So far we have dealt with only part of the story. Besides the integrin receptor binding to laminin, there are other cell–substrate adhesion molecules (Linnemann and Bock, 1989). One of these is cytotactin, which binds to a proteoglycan, a molecule made of protein and sugars. Cytotactin can take part in cell–cell adhesion as well. It is present on glial cells, whereas the cytotactin-binding proteoglycan is present in neurons. Cytotactin is found particularly on the pathways along which neurons are likely to migrate. Antibodies to cytotactin prevent neurons from migrating along these expected pathways. The adhesion of migrating neurons to guiding glial cells depends on the level of extracellular calcium, which can therefore act as a regulatory mechanism.

Another group of proteins found in cell membranes are the cell–cell adhesion molecules. Those that depend on calcium are called cadherins. N-Cadherin is present on all nerve cells, but only at points of cell–cell contact. N-Cadherin spans the cell membrane, the extracellular part binding to N-Cadherin molecules on other neurons and the intracellular part binding (via a linker protein called vinculin) to actin. N-Cadherin therefore resembles integrin in joining a point of external adhesion to the actin microfilaments in the intracellular cytoskeleton. It is unlike integrin in that (1) it binds only to other cells and not to the extracellular matrix, and (2) it binds homophilically to another N-Cadherin molecule, whereas integrin binds heterophilically to laminin.

Two more cell adhesion molecules, 'nerve cell adhesion molecule' (NCAM) and 'nerve growth factor-induced large external glycoprotein!' (NILE) differ from N-Cadherin in that they do not depend on calcium for their adhesive activity. The NCAM is an integral membrane protein which binds homophilically to NCAM molecules on other cells. It allows neurons to bind to other neurons and to astrocytes. Typically, it is present on cells that have not yet migrated. The levels of NCAM drop when cells are migrating, suggesting that they cannot migrate if they are still bound by it to other cells. Once migration is complete, however, NCAM genes are turned on again and NCAM reappears at points of contact between cells. It is also present in growth cone membranes, where it is responsible for a process called fasciculation. Early pathfinding fibres pioneer a route to a target then later fibres follow this path by growing along the pioneers. Thus bundles of fibres are formed, and NCAM is responsible for this. Interference with NCAM prevents the later fibres from following the pathfinders, and the ordered pattern of axonal growth is disrupted.

The last adhesion molecule we will mention is NILE. Like NCAM and integrin, it belongs to the immunoglobulin superfamily. It allows neurons to bind homophilically to each other, and perhaps heterophilically to glial cells, although this is less certain. It can also bind to extracellular matrix molecules such as fibronectin, which it resembles. It is involved in the outgrowth of neurites and the adhesion of later fibres to earlier pathfinders. As its unwieldy name suggests, it has the rather interesting property of being induced by growth factors, of which more later.

The main purpose of this section was to indicate that there are several molecules involved in the adhesion of nerve cells to each other, to glia and to the extracellular matrix. Some of these molecules bind only to themselves, some bind to other molecules. Some depend on calcium for their actions, some are independent of calcium. Some aid cell migration, some prevent it. Some help neurites to form bundles, some do not. Between them, these molecules are responsible, first, for directing the migration of neurons into layers; second, for signalling the pathways along which their neurites grow; and, third, for forming the connections between neurons. Their importance to neuronal development and redevelopment is hard to overestimate. The structure of the brain is determined by the dynamic redistribution of these molecules.

8.1.3 Growth factors

Extracellular molecules such as laminin and fibronectin were discussed in the section on the formation of new connections. These molecules, when bound to the extracellular matrix, are capable of inducing the formation of neurites and as such they are called neurotropic or neurite-promoting factors (NPF). They lose their neurotropic properties when they become soluble, unbound to the extracellular matrix. Another group of extracellular molecules are, by contrast, usually found in a soluble, unbound form. These soluble factors are responsible for maintaining the survival of neurons and their processes. They are called neurotrophic factors (note the 'h'), and they are distinct from neurotropic factors although they sometimes share the same properties. Several neurotrophic factors (NTF) have now been found, including brain-derived growth factor, ciliary ganglion derived-growth factor and the most famous of all, the original nerve growth factor (NGF).

Nerve growth factor is synthesized in the cells to be innervated and binds to receptors on the innervating neurons. Locally, it has a dual action. First, it induces nearby neurites to sprout. Second, it maintains the existence of neurites. As a neurite approaches its target, the target begins to synthesize NGF which, in turn, induces the neurite to express receptors for NGF. By inducing sprouts and then maintaining them, NGF appears to match innervation density to the size of the innervated

target. This is obviously as important in development and redevelopment as neurite induction and guidance.

The local action of NGF may be mediated partly by switching on Na^+–K^+ exchange pumps which pump potassium out of the neurite. In the absence of NGF, dependent neurites fail to expel potassium, and the rising internal concentration leads to retraction and death of the nerve process. Local effects of NGF are evident within minutes or hours and do not require the synthesis of new proteins.

In addition to local effects, NGF has long-term effects, evident within days. These require internalization of the growth factor bound to its receptor, followed by retrograde transport of the whole receptor–growth factor complex to the cell body, where it influences gene expression and hence the synthesis of the new proteins that mediate its long-term effects. Sympathetic neurons, developing dorsal root ganglion cells and the basal forebrain cholinergic neurons implicated in Alzheimer's disease are all dependent on NGF. Presumably other neurons are dependent on different growth factors.

8.1.4 Growth-associated proteins

The final point that we will consider in the formation of new connections is the role of growth-associated proteins (GAPs). One of them has many pseudonyms: B-50, GAP43, GAP48, F1, pp46, P-57. It is now established that all of these, discovered in different ways, are in fact one and the same protein. GAP43 establishes, better than any other evidence, the underlying identity of development, learning and regeneration because it plays a vital part in all three. Indeed, GAP43 has so many names precisely because it was repeatedly rediscovered by several scientists working independently in these superficially different fields.

GAP43 is present at high levels during the perinatal period of greatest neuronal development. Thereafter it decreases from most regions of the brain, but reappears whenever there is regeneration. In those brain regions involved most directly in learning and memory, however, GAP43 remains at high levels throughout adult life, suggesting that these regions retain some of the characteristics of developing brain. Like most other proteins, it is synthesized in the cell body. Rapid axonal transport carries it down to the growth cone where it is found in its highest concentrations either associated with the growth cone membrane or, to a lesser extent, in the vesicle from which the cone membrane will be formed. In adult nerurons GAP43 is confined to the immediately presynaptic membrane. GAP43 binds to a protein called calmodulin, a calcium-binding protein.

Before we can go further into the actions of GAP43, we need to take a detour into the molecular biology of cell signalling. By now the reader will be familiar with the concept of neurotransmitters binding to receptors which then activate G-proteins. G-proteins in their turn activate enzymes. One of these enzymes is phospholipase C, an enzyme which breaks up a fatty molecule bearing phosphate groups. In the present case, the fatty molecule is phosphatidyl inositol bisphosphate. Let us dissect this molecule.

Long chains of carbon with hydrogen atoms attached are known as acyl groups, or fatty acid chains. Two such chains linked to glycerol (antifreeze) form a molecule called diacylglycerol. Diacylglycerol linked to a sugar called inositol, which then has two phosphate groups attached to it, forms the molecule that we have been dissecting, phosphatidyl inositol bisphosphate.

Back to the G-protein-mediated activation of phospholipase C. Phospholipase C splits phosphatidyl inositol bisphosphate into two components. One component is diacylglycerol. The other component is inositol tri-phosphate. It is worth the effort of comprehending this complexity because the conversion of phosphatidyl inositol bisphosphate into diacylglycerol and inositol triphosphate lies at the heart, not only of many neuronal second messenger systems, but of many other cell signalling processes in biology, including development.

It has been mentioned briefly that calcium can be stored intracellularly in part of the endoplasmic reticulum, called the calcium-sequestering compartment. Inositol triphosphate moves to the calcium-sequestering compartment and opens its gates, the calcium ionophores, and calcium floods into the cytoplasm. In conjunction with diacylglycerol, raised intracellular calcium levels induce another enzyme, protein kinase C, to move to the cell membrane. This translocation of protein kinase C to the cell membrane is an essential step in the action of growth factors.

Now we can return to GAP43 which, you may remember, is closely associated with the cell membrane. Once protein kinase C has been translocated to the cell membrane it is in a position to catalyse the addition of a phosphate group to GAP43. Phosphorylated GAP43 is less able to bind to calmodulin, the calcium-binding protein with which it is normally associated. The rise in intracellular calcium caused by the action of inositol triphosphate also induces GAP43 to dissociate from calmodulin.

Calmodulin is therefore released in locally high concentration near the membrane of the growth cone. There, it binds to calcium, which activates it. Activated calmodulin causes an increase in phosphorylation of several proteins. One of these, tau protein, is involved in stabilizing microtubules. Another, fodrin, alters the way in which actin cross-links to itself and anchors to the cell membrane.

Meanwhile, the raised intracellular calcium levels have other actions. Calcium increases the interaction of myosin with actin, generating tension. Calcium increases the fusion of vesicles with the cell membrane, expanding it. Calcium encourages the dissociation of the cytoskeleton. These effects, coupled to the actions of calmodulin, combine in a complex biochemical interplay influencing the way in which growth cones form, change direction and elongate the neurite.

To summarize: growth-modulating agents act on receptors which induce G-protein to activate phospholipase C. Phospholipase C splits inositol triphosphate and diacylglycerol from phosphatidyl inositol bisphosphate. Inositol triphosphate releases calcium from intracellular stores and the released calcium, in concert with diacylglycerol, translocate protein kinase C to the cell membrane. Translocated protein kinase C phosphorylates GAP43 and that, together with the raised intracellular calcium, causes GAP43 to release calmodulin. Calmodulin binds to calcium, which causes it to induce the phosphorylation of tau protein and fodrin. Tau protein is involved in stabilizing microtubules and fodrin affects the linkage of actin to itself and to the cell membrane. Raised intracellular calcium triggers the interaction of myosin and actin, induces an expansion of the cell membrane by fusion of the vesicles and destabilizes the cytoskeleton. The net effect of this maelstrom of interlinked biochemical cascades is that neurites change direction and grow longer.

8.1.5 Other growth-modulating agents

We have just seen how G-proteins link receptors to the enzyme phospholipase C. G-proteins also activate another enzyme called adenylate cyclase. This enzyme converts adenosine triphosphate into the second messenger cyclic adenosine monophosphate (cAMP). A rise in cAMP has different effects in different neurons and in different species, but among these is a decrease in growth cone motility, an increase in microtubule polymerization, variable changes in neurite outgrowth and the formation of synapses. One of its effects is to induce the movement of organelles from the central part of the growth cone towards the lamellipodia, contributing to the maturation of a growth cone into a neurite.

Neurotransmitters also play a role in the growth of neurites. Some promote neuritic growth while others inhibit it. Neurotransmitters are released from growth cones and, conversely, act on growth cones, even before mature synapses are formed. In this context they probably act on G-proteins and phospholipase C or adenylate cyclase. It is probable that growth cones detect the appropriate balance of growth-enhancing and growth-inhibiting neurotransmitters and this might tell them when they have arrived at their targets. By finding out which transmitters have what effects in different systems, and then selectively encouraging or discouraging the relevant circuits, therapists may be able to influence the processes of neuritic elongation and growth cone arrest.

Finally, mention should be made of the effects of electric potential differences. There are currents entering the tips of filopodia and leaving their bases, but these currents are too weak to be of much significance. Experimentally, though, it can be shown that externally applied voltages have an influence on growth. The receptors for neurotropic and neurotrophic factors are proteins embedded in the semiliquid cell membrane. These proteins are usually charged molecules, so that when an external voltage is applied, the proteins migrate towards the cathode. The receptors concentrate on the cathodal side of a growth cone where they are available for adhesion to the extracellular matrix. Once adhesion occurs, growth follows in that direction. Externally applied voltages can therefore influence the direction of growth in much the same way that NGF influences the distribution of NILE. Perhaps this will provide an avenue for therapeutic intervention in regeneration of the damaged nervous system.

8.2 Increasing synaptic effectiveness

So far we have dealt only with making new connections. It is time to turn our attention to increasing the effectiveness of connections that already exist. Although long-term potentiation of synapses, described in the previous chapter, is not a perfect model of memory, it is probably the best cellular model currently available. It will be used here to illustrate changes in synaptic effectiveness.

The effectiveness of a synapse can be increased for at least three durations, lasting seconds and minutes, hours and days, or months and years (Matthies, 1989). These are sometimes called short-term, intermediate-term and long-term memory. Such changes can take place at three cellular locations: the presynaptic terminal, the postsynaptic membrane and the postsynaptic nucleus.

8.2.1 Presynaptic and short-term changes

During routine, low-frequency transmission across a synapse the transmembranous ionic exchanges are limited in extent and rapidly reversed by ionic pumps. With discharge rates high enough to induce long-term potentiation, however, the ionic changes are greater. In particular, voltage differences across the presynaptic membrane induced by the influx of sodium cause the voltage-gated calcium ionophores to open to a greater extent than usual. Calcium enters the presynaptic bouton in higher concentrations. This causes the translocation of protein kinase C to the presynaptic membrane, where it phosphorylates GAP43. Phosphorylation of GAP43 induces a cascade of biochemical reactions, the net effect of which is a short-term increase in the fusion of transmitter vesicles to the presynaptic membrane and consequently an increase in the release of the excitatory amino acid transmitter, glutamate. Increased release of glutamate enhances the effectiveness of the potentiated synapse for periods not exceeding 1 h.

These presynaptic changes underlying short-term potentiation of synapses are very reminiscent of the molecular processes causing elongation of neurites. The principal difference is that here, increased vesicle fusion results predominantly in greater release of neurotransmitter, whereas in the growth cone it increases the incorporation of vesicle membrane into the neurite's membrane, expanding it. This difference is merely one of emphasis because, in fact, measurements show that one of the effects of increased synaptic efficiency is an increase in the size of the presynaptic bouton. This may be no more than a consequence of increased fusion of transmitter vesicles, or it may contribute to potentiation by increasing the surface from which subsequent vesicles can be released. Growth of new connections and potentiation of synapses evidently exploit the same cellular mechanisms.

8.2.2   Local postsynaptic and intermediate-term changes

To understand local postsynaptic changes we must first discuss subtypes of glutamate receptors. Ionophores (ion channels) can be operated either by the binding of a chemical signal if they are ligand-gated channels, or by changes in transmembrane potential if they are voltage-gated channels. One glutamate receptor subtype is a simple ligand-gated sodium channel called the quisqualate receptor. Arrival of glutamate opens the channel and allows the entry of sodium ions down their electrochemical gradient, evoking an excitatory postsynaptic potential.

A second glutamate receptor subtype is a more complicated channel for calcium, called the N-methyl D-aspartate (NMDA) receptor. On the one hand it conforms to a ligand-gated channel, in that it will not open unless glutamate binds to it. On the other hand, even when glutamate has bound to it, it remains blocked by magnesium ions when the potential difference across the membrane is close to resting levels. If, however, the membrane is partially depolarized, magnesium is driven from the channel orifice and calcium can enter. The NMDA channel is therefore a ligand-gated but voltage-modulated channel. Only the simultaneous binding of glutamate to the receptor and the concurrent depolarization of the membrane via a neighbouring channel will operate it. This has been likened to the association of conditioned and unconditioned stimuli, the latter exciting the quisqualate receptor and the former exciting the NMDA receptor.

We will now investigate how glutamate receptors contribute to local postsynaptic potentiation. Under non-potentiating conditions low-frequency transmission, analogous to unconditioned stimulation, releases enough glutamate to bind NMDA and quisqualate receptors. The quisqualate chan-

nels open, but because there is only a moderate quantity of glutamate bound to them, they open only sufficiently to allow the entry of sodium in quantities that generate normal postsynaptic evoked potentials, but no more. Because the postsynaptic potential changes are only moderate, the NMDA channel remains blocked by magnesium.

Higher frequency stimulation, analogous to conditioned stimulation, releases sufficient glutamate to open quisqualate channels to a greater degree. More sodium enters than before and the resulting postsynaptic potentials are greater, as expected with temporal or spatial summation. Glutamate also binds to NMDA receptors, but this time the degree of depolarization is sufficient to drive magnesium from the channel, and the NMDA channel is fully opened. Calcium rushes in through the NMDA channel and binds to calmodulin held in the postsynaptic web visible just deep to the postsynaptic membrane in electron micrographs. Calmodulin bound to calcium activates protein kinase C and the latter enzyme phosphorylates the quisqualate receptor.

The exact nature of the consequences of this last step are not yet determined, but several intermediate-term changes are possible. Phosphorylated quisqualate receptors may have greater affinity for glutamate, binding it more effectively. They may acquire the ability to open more often, or they may stay open longer. Alternatively, some quisqualate receptor molecules that may have been kept in a previously unresponsive state may now become responsive to glutamate. Any of these changes would then enhance subsequent responses to the presynaptic release of a given quantity of glutamate.

Whatever the exact nature of the final step, there is an increased effectiveness of the potentiated synapse. This local potentiation has several characteristics. First, it lasts for a matter of hours, not seconds or weeks. Second, this potentiation can be induced in dendrites even after they have been cut off from their cell bodies. Third, no synthesis of new proteins is required, since all the changes involve the modification of proteins that are already present in the local postsynaptic region.

8.2.3   Nuclear and long-term changes

The previous two sets of changes are interesting and may account for short- and intermediate-term storage, but they are not responsible for the memories that can last a life-time. Genuinely long-term changes always involve the synthesis of new proteins, and they affect the nucleus of the postsynaptic cell.

High-frequency stimulation, or conditioned learning, result in the activation of receptor-linked second messenger systems that induce the phosphorylation of regulatory proteins. These phosphorylated regulatory proteins subsequently enter the postsynaptic cell's nucleus where they induce the transcription of a set of genes soon after learning takes place. This set of genes is transcribed to RNA which moves into the cell to be translated into protein. The proteins formed in this first wave of gene expression are small, soluble proteins. They are the products of master regulatory genes, called proto-oncogenes, and their function is to turn on whole families of genes coding for the proteins actually used in a particular cellular process. Soon after learning, these soluble proteins disappear, but only after they have initiated the transcription of a second set of genes.

Transcription and translation of the second set of genes begins some hours after a task is learned. The proteins coded by this second set of genes are large and insoluble. After being synthesized by the ribosomes attached to the granular endoplasmic reticulum, they migrate by dendritic transport back to the synapses whose activation led to their synthesis in the first place. Precisely what they do to these synapses is still the subject of research, but the net effect is a very long-term potentiation, lasting as much as a life-time. Perhaps these proteins ensure that their own synthesis is perpetuated, acting like a permanently turned on genetic switch. Perhaps they induce structural changes such as dendritic sprouting or enlargement of postsynaptic spines. Perhaps they are more efficient receptor molecules or more catalytic second messenger enzymes. Whatever their mechanism, it is known for certain that they are essential to long-term memory. Without them, information can be stored for no more than a few hours at most. They represent a permanent change in phenotype and they are the molecules that enable us to learn and remember.

8.3 Concluding remarks

This chapter has been an attempt to introduce therapists to the molecular and cellular details underlying developmental growth and mnemonic changes in synaptic efficiency. For the sake of clarity, anatomical changes have been emphasized in the section on development and biochemical changes in the section on synaptic potentiation. This difference is no more than the result of selectively focusing attention on different aspects of similar phenomena. The anatomical changes in growth are brought about by biochemical changes very similar to those involved in learning and synaptic potentiation. Conversely, learning has been repeatedly shown to involve anatomical changes, such as increases in the size and number of presynaptic boutons and postsynaptic spines, increased length and increased branching of dendrites, and migration of presynaptic terminals. The only real difference between learning and development is that the latter is brought about by the phylogenetic experience of an individual's ancestors whereas the former is the result of the individual's own experience. Otherwise they involve the same receptors, the same second messenger systems, the same kinases and phosphorylases, and the same morphological changes. Learning is only a redevelopment of an already existing nervous system, whereas development creates a nervous system that does not previously exist. Regeneration after injury combines features of both. Successful therapies must learn the trick of inducing the redevelopment of damaged nervous systems. If they work, they will operate via the molecular and cellular mechanisms outlined in this chapter, or by equivalent processes.

References

Linnemann, D. and Bock, E. (1989) Cell adhesion molecules in neural development. *Dev. Neurosci.* **11**: 149–73.

Matthies, H. (1989) In search of cellular mechanisms of memory. *Progress in Neurobiology* **32**: 277–349.

Mitchison, T. and Kirschner, M. (1988) Cytoskeletal dynamics and nerve growth. *Neuron* **1**: 761–72.

Van Hooff, C. O. M., Oestreicher, A. B., De Graan, P. N. E. and Gispen, W. H. (1989) Role of the growth cone in neuronal differentiation. *Molecular Neurobiology* **3**: 101–33.

Chapter 9

A critical review of contemporary therapies

9.1 Introduction

The aim of rehabilitation is to restore an individual's ability to function in the environment. Habilitation involves developing an ability not previously held by the individual. Following damage to the central nervous system (CNS) adults require rehabilitating in order to restore them to their previous level of function. The arguments presented in this book so far lead us to suggest that if neurologically damaged adults are to achieve the maximum effect of rehabilitation in the long-term then the ability of the CNS to adapt following damage must be exploited and guided. When damage occurs to the CNS in young babies and in children then the individual has not reached the full potential of adulthood and therefore the CNS needs to be assisted in developing that potential. To enable a patient to develop or to be restored to full potential, plastic changes to enhance normal movement must be encouraged. If plastic adaptation to abnormal movement is allowed then in the long-term the abnormal movement will become more established and function will decrease. Therefore the aim of rehabilitation will be lost. The therapies need to be able to:

1. Strengthen normal synaptic chains and neuronal sets.
2. Guide axonal sprouting.
3. Facilitate unmasking of alternative or previously subservient pathways in the CNS in order to maintain normal function through alternate routes.

To return to 'classical' stimulus response physiology; what goes in determines what comes out in the short-term. However, the ability of the CNS to adapt its structure to suit the required function means that what goes in modifies the inside so that it can more easily give the same response in the future. So abnormal movement in the short-term will reinforce abnormal movement in the long-term by making it easier for the CNS to respond to the same stimulus in the future. In the main, therapies used to rehabilitate brain-damaged patients are based on stimulus response physiology but the response is always reinforced whether it is normal or abnormal. A knowledge of stimulus response is necessary in order to appreciate the basis for the therapies but a knowledge of plastic adaptation alters our understanding of their effect and therefore determines their future development.

This chapter will present a brief history of therapeutic approaches to rehabilitation of CNS dysfunction and a critique of contemporary therapies. The critique will be based on the ability of the therapies to guide plastic adaptation in the CNS in order to achieve, restore or maintain normal movement and function in the long-term. Finally this chapter will present a guide for effective therapeutic intervention based on the concepts presented in this book.

9.2 A history of the approach to neurological rehabilitation

The traditional approach to the rehabilitation of the brain-injured patient was to concentrate on remaining abilities. So, in a patient with hemiplegia due to a stroke affecting one hemisphere, treatment aimed to improve functional abilities by use of the unaffected side only. To aid walking the affected leg was replaced by a three-legged stick, called a tripod and the goal of treatment, as stated by Perry (1969) was the 'attainment of a safe, not a normal, mode of travel'. This approach had obvious limitations both aesthetically and functionally. Many activities are impossible unless normal movement can be retrained in the affected limbs; for example, such activities as unscrewing the lid from a jar and peeling potatoes are impossible unless normal movement is retrained in the affected arm and hand. Also, while the use of a tripod or walking stick may aid walking in the short-term, because the gait pattern is abnormal and involves moving the affected leg in a spastic pattern, the spasticity is encouraged and reinforced (see below). In the long-term this then leads to a reduction in function because of increased spasticity.

In this traditional approach, if any attempt was made to rehabilitate the affected limbs then the inability to move was treated as a lower motoneuron disorder. That is, if a patient with spasticity in the flexor muscles of the upper limb could not extend his or her elbow this was considered to be a weakness of the triceps muscle and appropriate strengthening exercises were given. However, current concepts of movement control and the disturbance in spasticity suggest that the triceps muscle is prevented from moving the elbow either due to excessive co-contraction in the spastic biceps or due to excessive reciprocal inhibition in the triceps. The triceps will only be able to extend the elbow if the spasticity in the biceps is reduced, therefore also reducing any excessive co-contraction in biceps and any excessive reciprocal inhibition in the triceps. Also in the traditional approach calipers or braces were used to support a 'weak' leg (see Perry, 1969). If the weakness is caused by spasticity and its effects then an attempt to relieve the spasticity in the first instance would seem a more positive approach. So the relief of spasticity would seem to be the main criterion on which the treatment of these patients should be based.

Equally, in patients with other symptoms of CNS damage such as ataxia, a restoration of function was achieved by this early approach to rehabilitation by making use of remaining abilities or by the use of walking aids or other mechanical aids to function. If a patient had defective balance reactions in trunk and lower limbs then he was given a walking frame to aid walking. The four-legged walking frame allowed patients to move from place to place albeit in an abnormal pattern and removed the necessity of trunk and lower limb balance reactions. Once given a walking frame patients had no need to redevelop these balance reactions.

While this approach to rehabilitation may seem short-sighted now, it was a great advance in the 1940s. Before the Second World War rehabilitation of brain-injured patients was almost non-existent and patients were left to lie in bed. This produced its own problems. Consequently, the development of the traditional approach was hailed as a great innovation and it has taken a long time for it to be relinquished. Some elements still exist today.

In the 1950s, new physiologically based approaches to the rehabilitation of brain-injured patients began to be developed (Bobath, 1963; Brunnstrom, 1961, 1970; Fay, 1948, 1954; Kabat, 1952; Rood, 1956). These approaches were based on empirical observation and clinical experience as well as on current neurophysiological concepts and they all attempted to restore a patient to 'normality'. In many cases (e.g. the Bobath approach) the concept was developed from observation alone and a suitable theory was adopted to explain the effects. However, many of the observations were ahead of the physiological thinking of that time and therefore their proponents found difficulty in finding acceptance.

Many of the approaches made use of peripheral input (either cutaneous or proprioceptive) to facilitate or modify motor output. The proprioceptive neuromuscular facilitation (PNF) approach, as described by Kabat (1952), uses various types of afferent input to facilitate movement, including input from the muscle spindles caused by stretch of the muscle or by a resisted voluntary contraction. When using the PNF approach, mass or total movement patterns are used wherever possible rather than exercises that involve contractions of a single muscle group. It is suggested that as movements normally occur as a pattern of activity in different muscle groups then this should be encouraged. The approach developed by Rood (1956) also makes use of peripheral input, particularly cutaneous stimulation. The approach developed by Bobath (1963), firstly for the treatment of cerebral palsied children, makes use of the facilitation of normal postural reflex activity (*sic*) to provide a base for, and therefore facilitate, normal movement. Bobath first observed that altering the position of proximal joints could alter muscle tone throughout a limb. This was later developed to a movement of proximal joints, preferably an active movement by the patient. It was felt that normal movement (particularly of proximal joints and the trunk) gave a normal peripheral input to the CNS and therefore facilitated further normal movement. These approaches, particularly when used to treat brain-damaged children, also made use of developmental sequences of movement, encouraging the development of normal movement in the correct sequence seen in normal children. Many of these approaches are therefore often referred to as neuro-developmental approaches.

While Bobath tried to facilitate normal movement patterns and inhibit abnormal patterns, both Fay and Brunnstrom advocated the use of mass flexion and extension synergies which would be considered abnormal in anyone other than a very young baby. Fay (1948) refers to the flexion and extension synergies as patterned movements and the reflexes which are released following cortical lesions, such as the flexor withdrawal reflex, extensor thrust and tonic neck reflexes as 'basic reflexes of spinal automatism'. Fay felt that eliciting these reflexes in children with cerebral palsy was a better form of treatment than passive movement alone. Brunnstrom (1961, 1970) made use of these mass synergies in the treatment of spastic hemiplegia following stroke. She considered the first goal in treatment to be for the patient to acquire the ability to perform the mass flexion and extension synergies of hemiplegia. She felt that these synergies are the stepping stones for more advanced work and that they can be considerably modified. Various types of peripheral stimulation were suggested as useful in modifying these basic synergies.

At this point controversy was already developing with regard to the use of abnormal movement patterns. Some workers in the field felt that abnormal movement should never be allowed. Others felt that patients had to go through the stages of recovery following brain damage and that this involved the stage of abnormal or primitive movement. Therefore the abnormal movement was encouraged.

All these approaches as they developed through the 1950s and the 1960s involved treating either children or adults with brain damage for an hour or so per day or even every other day, although most encouraged the continuation of the treatment at home by parents or carers or in school by teachers. In the 1960s the Peto approach to managing brain-damaged children came to the fore. This method, referred to as conductive education, uses a neuropsychological approach rather than a neurophysiological approach. The method uses techniques based on learning theory to reinforce motor learning by the brain-damaged child and the aim is to educate neurologically damaged children so that they are able to fit physical, psychological and social norms (see Todd, 1990) and therefore function in society. The approach was developed in Hungary by Professor Peto and is still most fully and widely implemented in that country. The approach has now been introduced into the UK and is also used in the management of adult hemiplegic stroke patients. The Peto approach differs from other approaches in its emphasis on continuous (24 h) reinforcement to ensure that learning takes place. In other words this approach is encouraging plastic adaptation to new motor activities and also social and functional activities. It therefore provides the final key to unlock the remaining door to successful rehabilitation.

9.3 Therapeutic intervention in spasticity: guiding plastic adaptation

The development and treatment of spasticity can serve as an example of plastic adaptation within the CNS. Spasticity may develop because of inappropriate adaptation of the CNS but handling techniques may be able to guide the adaptation to make it more normal and therefore to improve function in the long-term. Arguments for the causes of spasticity and for approaches to its management and treatment will now be presented.

Spasticity involves multiple phenomena including hyperreflexia and abnormal (mass) movement patterns, and is seen in patients with damage to ventromedial and dorsolateral descending pathways (see Chapter 6, Section 6.5) from the brain to the spinal cord. The hyperreflexia leads to an increased resistance to passive movement and there is also an inability to perform movement patterns in opposition to the spastic patterns due to inappropriate co-contraction in the spastic muscles and/or excessive reciprocal inhibition in their antagonists. The fact that the increased passive stretch responses may be abolished by drug therapy while the inappropriate co-contraction during active movement remains (McLellan and Hassan, 1982) suggests that the phenomena are not all due to the same cause, although all may be due to a general disinhibition of the spinal cord.

Current theories on the mechanisms underlying spasticity suggest that the increased passive stretch responses are due to an increase in the tonic stretch reflex (TSR). This TSR is a polysynaptic spinal reflex and in a normal relaxed subject it is not evident on passive movement. In a normal subject the reflex is seen when a muscle is stretched during a voluntary contraction, i.e. in the presence of alpha and gamma co-activation, and it is thought to provide a reflex alteration in force of muscle contraction in order to overcome any resistance to the voluntary movement. Alpha–gamma co-activation enables the muscle spindle to respond even when the extrafusal muscle fibres are contracting and therefore unloading the spindle and so the response to stretch or resistance remains as long as the stretch remains (it is a tonic reflex). The TSR thus produced reinforces alpha-motoneuron activity when needed. The size of the response to the stretch is determined by the velocity of the passive stretch and also by the force of the voluntary contraction already in operation. In patients with spasticity, the TSR has been shown to be in a fully 'switched-on' or hyperactive state at all times (Neilson, 1972) so that it can be elicited by passive stretch alone without any concomitant voluntary contraction. The hyperactivity may be presumed to be due to an increase in spindle sensitivity due to an increase in fusimotor activity or to a disinhibition of spinal pathways associated with the reflex.

Classical theories of spasticity attributed the phenomena to an increased fusimotor drive but Burke (1980, 1988) argues that there is no evidence of increased fusimotor activity in spastic patients. However, there is evidence of a disinhibition of spinal pathways as shown by the inability of spastic subjects to suppress the tonic vibration reflex (TVR). The TVR is a tonic reflex muscle contraction caused by vibration of muscle spindles which induces activity in Ia afferents independent of fusimotor activity (Eklund and Hagbarth, 1966). Normal subjects can voluntarily suppress the TVR and when they do this there is no sign of a decrease in muscle spindle discharge (Burke *et al.*, 1976) suggesting they are suppressing or inhibiting spinal reflex pathways. Patients with spasticity are unable to suppress the TVR suggesting an inability to suppress spinal pathways associated with the TVR.

Presynaptic inhibition, an important mechanism in controlling activity in spinal pathways, is one of the inhibitory mechanisms that appears to be disturbed in spasticity. In the cat and in humans the TVR has been shown to abolish the phasic monosynaptic reflex while it is activated and it

appears to do this by presynaptic inhibition (Gilles *et al.*, 1969; Dindar and Verrier, 1975; Ashby and Verrier, 1980). In spastic hemiplegia in humans, the suppression of the monosynaptic reflex by vibration is reduced and in spinal humans it is absent (Burke and Lance, 1973; Ashby *et al.*, 1980), thus suggesting a loss of presynaptic inhibitory mechanisms in spasticity. In 1989, Nance *et al.* were able to show that the administration of clonidine increased vibratory inhibition of the monosynaptic reflex (measured by the H-reflex) in spinal cord-injured patients. This suggests that the ingestion of clonidine which is an alpha-2-adrenergic agonist is switching on presynaptic inhibitory mechanisms. In experiments on acute spinal cats it was the switching on of these adrenergic terminals by clonidine or dopa which led to the initiation of stepping patterns and also these terminals are implicated in the control of short-latency flexor reflexes and the activation of the long-latency reflexes thought to be involved in stepping (see Chapter 6, Sections 6.5 and 6.6). These adrenergic descending pathways may be very important in the inhibitory control of spinal pathways to allow for normal movement and part or all of their action may be presynaptic.

When damage occurs suddenly to descending pathways to the spinal cord it is followed by a period of spinal shock. Only after a period of days or weeks may spasticity appear. This has led to a consideration of spasticity as a phenomenon of plasticity rather than of release. If spasticity was due simply to a release of spinal pathways from higher centres then it should appear immediately following a lesion. However, it has been shown (Ashby and Verrier, 1980) that vibratory inhibition of the monosynaptic reflex is increased in the paralysed limbs in the early stages after the lesion. Only in long-standing lesions is it found to be less than normal. On this basis it has been suggested that spasticity may be due to plastic rearrangement in the CNS. Also, studies in the cat have suggested that following spinal cord hemisection leading to a loss of descending pathways there is a recovery of function which could not be attributed simply to spared segmental afferent input as it does not appear immediately. The recovery takes several weeks and is attributed to sprouting of segmental afferent fibres in order to enhance activity and replace lost descending fibres (see Goldberger and Murray, 1988). In spasticity caused by a lesion to descending pathways collateral sprouting could lead to an increase in facilitatory connections from the periphery causing hyperreflexia. During the development of spasticity presynaptic inhibition may be lost or the amount present may become insufficient. Burke (1988) argues that plastic changes and a release phenomenon may occur together as plastic adaptation could not occur without the release.

It has been suggested that supraspinal presynaptic inhibition, controlling spinal reflex activity and therefore movement, is subserved in intact animals by a segmental presynaptic inhibition which comes mainly from proximal regions of the limbs (Lundberg, 1979). The control of incoming pain information to the spinal cord is also suggested as being due to a segmental and a supraspinal presynaptic inhibition as well as probably by a postsynaptic inhibition. It has been possible to control pain through stimulation of large diameter afferents by acupuncture or by electrical stimulation and equally it has been shown empirically that movement and muscle tone in a limb can be controlled through manipulation of proximal limb regions (Bobath, 1990). Input through 'correct' movement of proximal regions may be able to switch on and reinforce segmental presynaptic inhibition so that it can take over from lost supraspinal influences. Wall (1980) described the process of unmasking as a phenomenon of plasticity. Unmasking takes place when synapses which normally subserve an activity in the intact animal take over the function when the dominant pathway is lost. Wall and Werman (1976) carried out a study into the activity in dorsal horn cells of the rat. They found that some cells in the dorsal horn received connections from segmental afferents and also from more long-ranging afferents. Further studies showed that in the intact animal the cells did not show any response to stimulation of long-range afferents but they responded to the segmental afferents. After lesioning of the segmental afferents, and following electrical or natural stimulation of the long-range afferents, the cells showed a response (Devor *et al.*, 1977). It was suggested that in the intact animal the long-range afferents were inhibited by the segmental afferents. Once the segmental afferents were lost they became disinhibited or unmasked and were able to take over the function they subserved (see Fig. 9.1). The important point to note is that the subserving pathways will only be made permanent if stimulation is applied over a period of time. Segmental presynaptic inhibitory connections may subserve supraspinal presynaptic inhibitory connections and

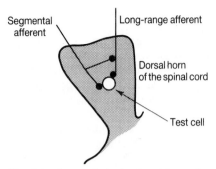

Fig. 9.1 Some cells in the dorsal horn of the spinal cord of the rat receive connections from segmental afferents and also from more long-ranging afferents. In the intact animal the cells do not respond to the long-range afferents but they do respond to the segmental afferents. After lesioning of the segmental afferents the cells respond to a stimulation of the long-range afferents. This suggests that in the intact animal the long-range afferents are inhibited by the segmental afferents but when disinhibited or unmasked they are able to take over the function they subserved.

in the case of supraspinal loss they may be able to take over. This is supported by empirical observations of the use of movement of proximal limb joints to reduce tone in the limbs. However, this effect would not become permanent unless the connections are stressed over a period of time. This points to a need for therapies to use manipulations that will 'switch on' presynaptic inhibition, probably through stimulation of proximal regions, but they need to do this over a period of time. Plastic changes in skeletal muscle only occurred if the nerve to the muscle was stimulated using the correct trophic code for several hours a day for 30–40 days (Kidd *et al.*, 1989). If natural peripheral stimulation leads to a normal movement then it must also be providing a correct trophic code to reinforce synaptic connections for the movement by the release of neuromodulators at the synaptic cleft. However, once the patient is left to his own devices he may revert to the use of abnormal movement patterns. If these abnormal movements are being used for the greater part of the day then these are the ones that will be reinforced. The reinforcement of normal movement will only occur if the normal peripheral input occurs for a sufficient period of time each day.

Because spasticity is also thought to be due to plastic adaptation through axonal sprouting, treatment also needs to be directed at preventing or guiding the axonal sprouting so that it leads to a facilitation of 'normal' synaptic pathways. This could best be done while the plastic adaptation is taking place immediately after a lesion. It has been shown that axonal sprouting can be guided or enhanced through electrical stimulation in rats (Maehlen and Arid, 1982). Also homotypic sprouting is suggested as having a competitive advantage in the spinal cord (see Goldberger and Murray, 1988) so any remaining parts of the same system may be more likely to sprout and recover lost synapses. Therefore, the possibility of aiding homotypic sprouting and recovering more normal movement should be greater. Aiding homotypic sprouting through normal peripheral input or through electrical stimulation could prevent the development of extra facilitatory connections and lead to the recovery of the lost inhibition.

9.4 Contemporary therapeutic approaches in disorders of the central nervous system

Attempts have been made to determine the effectiveness of contemporary therapeutic approaches to rehabilitation of brain-injured patients through experimental research methodology. Most attempts have involved a clinical trial approach whereby one group of patients are administered the treatment under review and another group of patients either act as a control or receive a different treatment. This approach has many deficiencies. The methodology requires an homogenous group of patients for each group and a standardized treatment approach. Both are virtually impossible as patients are all different depending on the site and extent of their lesion and treatments are tailored to suit each individual patient. Even if these requirements are deemed to be met or are ignored, the question of measurement gives rise to further problems. Many researchers 'employ' therapists to undertake the treatment and they (the researchers themselves) decide on the measurements to be made to evaluate effectiveness. Often their idea of effectiveness is a short-term increase in a particular functional ability and this may be measured by using one of the scales developed for measuring activities of daily living (see Sheikh *et al.*, 1978). However, the therapists implementing the treatment may have as their goal the achievement of more normal movement patterns when performing the particular functions, in the hope that this will prevent further deterioration in the future. In order to determine whether or not this goal has been

achieved there is a need to measure quality of movement when performing the functional activity and also to measure in the long-term. For this reason it is necessary to develop methods by which quality of movement can be measured. The majority of current approaches to rehabilitation aim to achieve normal movement but even in evaluating individual patients none of them measure normal movement objectively. A more fundamental approach to the evaluation of rehabilitation may be to consider its physiological basis.

9.4.1 The facilitation of normal movement through handling

Many physiotherapeutic approaches attempt to facilitate normal movement by the use of afferent input from the periphery, the input being controlled by handling techniques. Bobath (1963, 1990) first observed that muscle tone in a limb could be altered in cerebral palsied children by altering the position of proximal joints. The proximal joints were moved into positions opposite to the spastic pattern and their positions became known as 'reflex-inhibiting positions' because they inhibited or reduced the abnormal hyperreflexia. Bobath later amended the term to that of 'reflex-inhibiting patterns' as movement of the joints into the positions was considered to have a greater effect than the maintenance of the position. The use of proximal limb regions to influence motor output from the spinal cord accords with the findings from animal studies into the neural control of locomotion (see Grillner, 1981). Movement of proximal limb regions may be helping descending pathways in the initiation and the modification of basic spinal programmes of movement or, in the case of complete loss of descending control, may be replacing them. Movement of proximal limb regions may also be switching on segmental presynaptic inhibitory mechanisms (see Lundberg, 1979) and so restoring normal inhibitory mechanisms necessary for normal movement.

The importance of correct hip alignment in normal gait in humans has also been observed, in both normal subjects and in adult stroke patients with a spastic hemiplegia. Herman *et al.* (1973) and Cook and Cozzens (1976) also emphasize the importance of loading and unloading the limb as well as the correct alignment of the trunk and pelvis for the initiation of gait in humans. Miller and Musa (1982) measured movements of the hip joint and limb loading in normal subjects and in stroke patients during gait. They found that movements of the hip joint in the sagittal plane in the affected leg of the stroke patients were significantly lower than normal subjects. Values for hip joint excursion were also compared by Miller and Musa to values obtained from a clinical assessment which measured quality of movement as well as functional ability (see Ashburn, 1982). There was a significant positive correlation between the measurements suggesting that a reduction in hip movement is associated with a reduction in the patient's functional and motor performance. In this study, limb loading was also significantly reduced in the affected leg of patients who use a walking stick or a tripod. Bobath has also emphasized the importance of correct limb loading and loading of proximal regions has been implicated in animal studies as being of similar importance to proximal joint movements (Grillner, 1981). If patients are allowed to use a walking stick or a tripod then they will tend to reduce loading on the affected leg in favour of the stick.

Bobath describes a situation of abnormal postural reflex activity in children with brain lesions (Bobath, 1971) and her approach was developed to retrain a normal postural reflex activity (*sic*). This is in line with the strictly hierarchical understanding of motor control by the CNS. Bobath was suggesting that automatic postural adjustments constitute a lower level in the hierarchy than voluntary movements intrinsic to the limb and that they are entirely reflex in nature, i.e. occurring in response to an external stimulus. Because they were considered to be at a lower level they therefore needed to be retrained first. While more modern approaches to the understanding of motor control may suggest parallel descending systems rather than a hierarchy and also postural adjustments that are not entirely reflex, it is still true that automatic postural adjustment must occur in combination with or immediately preceding voluntary movement of the limbs if overall movement is to be normal. Therefore attempts to facilitate these postural adjustments would seem reasonable. Automatic postural adjustments resulting in different distributions of postural tone (termed postural sets by Bobath) appear to be controlled by the ventromedial descending pathways (see Chapter 6, Section 6.5) and the region of the ventral horn of the spinal cord influenced by these pathways appears to be accessed by peripheral input from proximal limb regions and the trunk. Bobath refers to these regions as proximal key points of control whereby movement and tonus can be influenced distally (Bobath, 1990).

Because movement or change of position of proximal limb regions leads to an observable alteration in tone Bobath felt that different pathways were being opened up in the spinal cord depending on the position of the limb. She cited the observations of Magnus (1909) who observed that in chronic spinal dogs the initial position of a limb could determine its response to a knee tap applied to the contralateral limb and also the observations of Von Uexkull (1904) on the brittlestar. Magnus (1926) developed his shunting rule which states that:

> . . . the different attitudes with their different distribution of tone and tension in the numerous muscles of the body, are associated with different distributions of reflex irritability over the central nervous system. Therefore one and the same stimulus may cause quite different reflex reactions according to the different attitudes of the animal at the moment the stimulus is applied.

These observations of phase-dependent reflex reversal have now been supported by studies using modern physiological techniques (Forssberg *et al.*, 1975; Grillner and Rossignol, 1978; Rossignol and Gautier, 1980). Also the idea of movement or change in position of proximal limb regions opening or closing pathways in the CNS is strongly supported by the evidence of the wide convergence onto interneurons in the spinal cord from peripheral afferents and from descending tracts and the fact that pathways can be opened or closed by descending or peripheral effects.

More recently the Bobath approach has moved towards a greater emphasis on the trunk (the central key point) as the first key point of control having a greater influence on the whole body than the proximal (limb) key points. Through facilitation of the central and the proximal key points attempts are made to regulate muscle tone throughout the body. In the rehabilitation of adult hemiplegic patients much emphasis is now placed on the correct alignment of the key points in any particular postural set (e.g. sitting, standing). It is felt that if the patient has the correct alignment of the key points in a postural set such as sitting then the correct pathways in the CNS will be open, postural tonal distribution will be normal and the patient will be more easily able to move from the postural set to another such as standing. So the Bobath approach emphasizes the facilitation of normal movement and muscle tone by a normal input due to normal postural adjustments and movement. Evaluation of its effect on an individual patient is by a qualitative assessment of movement.

While the Bobath approach emphasizes normal movement and muscle tone as a basis for the reinforcement of normal movement, proprioceptive neuromuscular facilitation (PNF) emphasizes the use of peripheral and descending input to the spinal cord to reinforce existing output (alpha-motoneuron activity) (see Knott and Voss, 1969). This does not mean that PNF encourages abnormal movement but techniques are used to facilitate and guide the normal movement when it occurs. The PNF approach uses various types of peripheral input to facilitate and reinforce movement (Kabat, 1952). These include input from muscle spindles caused by applying stretch to a muscle or by resisting a voluntary contraction and also cutaneous input. Reinforcement of descending input from the brain is achieved by encouraging mass movement patterns rather than contractions of individual muscles and by encouraging maximum effort from the patient. This maximum effort is encouraged through guidance of the patient, improving motivation and making use of visual and auditory input to the cerebral cortex.

Encouraging mass patterns is thought to be a way of reinforcing movement because the cortex tends to direct patterns of movement rather than contraction of individual muscles but also when mass patterns are used it is suggested that there is an overflow from strong muscles to weak muscles. It is known that Ia afferent input from contracting muscles will facilitate alpha efferent activity to other muscles or muscle groups. This was first postulated by Eccles and Lundberg in 1958 from studies in the cat but has recently been confirmed in humans (Pierrot-Deseilligny *et al.*, 1981b; Forget *et al.*, 1989). Forget *et al.* (1989) demonstrated the facilitation of the quadriceps H-reflex by the stimulation of group Ia afferents from pretibial flexors both while the quadriceps was at rest and at the beginning of a voluntary contraction. However, the strength of the facilitation caused by a voluntary contraction of the pretibial flexors rather than an electrical stimulation of Ia afferents may be in doubt. Also, many other muscle groups need investigating before a comprehensive pattern of facilitation can be drawn up.

Another way in which PNF reinforces alpha-motoneuron activity is by the use of maximum voluntary contractions and maximal resistance. Inducing a maximum voluntary contraction from the patient and giving a maximum resistance would induce a maximal tonic stretch reflex effect (see Section 9.3). The tonic stretch reflex increases with the force of voluntary contraction and therefore encouraging a maximum contraction should ensure the greatest reinforcement as a result of resistance to the movement.

The approach developed by Rood is similar to that of PNF, as it attempts to facilitate movement by use of peripheral input to the spinal cord. Rood (1956) talks of the activation or inhibition of muscles through 'stimulation of specific sensory receptors'. So, like the PNF approach and the Bobath approach, Rood is attempting to be specific and to inhibit unwanted movement and facilitate wanted movement. Rood also emphasizes the need for normal reciprocal inhibition during a voluntary movement, a concept emphasized by Bobath and PNF proponents also. In particular, the use of cutaneous stimulation is advocated by Rood. It was demonstrated in 1954 by Eldred and Hagbarth that cutaneous stimulation reinforces alpha- and gamma-motoneuron activity in underlying muscles and inhibits more distal muscles. Pierrot-Deseilligny *et al.* (1981a) were able to show that in humans the inhibition of more distant muscles by cutaneous stimulation was due to Ib inhibitory effects.

These approaches (Bobath, Rood, PNF) all emphasize the facilitation of normal movement and the consideration of the whole person rather than movement at one joint. Also they advocate the use of 'movements' rather than 'exercises'. Carr and Shepherd (1989) base their motor learning theory on the assumption that the rehabilitation of brain-injured patients should be both task and context specific. They suggest that there will be little carry-over from 'exercises' into functional activity and so the rehabilitation should involve practice of tasks or 'functions'. This idea of carry-over is important if the effects of treatment interventions to retrain normal movement are to be effective in the long-term. In this respect the modern Bobath emphasis on normal movement for the reinforcement of normal movement, and the retraining of patients in this normal movement should be most effective. However, particularly in the early stages, carry-over may be limited.

9.4.2 The use of abnormal reflex activity

Unlike Bobath, Rood and advocates of PNF, Fay
(1948) and Brunnstrom (1961, 1970) advocate the
use of mass flexion and extension synergies which
would be considered abnormal in anyone other
than a young baby. The mass movement patterns
seen in a young baby are possible evidence of the
capability of the spinal cord to produce basic movement patterns. These patterns are modified by
descending input from the brain and the development of this ability begins immediately following
birth. In children with cerebral palsy there may be
motor delay and these basic patterns may exist for
longer or even indefinitely. Fay advocates their use
in rehabilitation. He feels that to elicit the reflexes
is a better form of therapy than passive movement
alone. However, passive movement through normal adult patterns may give a more appropriate
input to the spinal cord than the effect of abnormal
reflex activity. These abnormal or basic movement
patterns are also seen in adult patients following
CNS damage and the release of the spinal cord
from supraspinal influence. In the recovery of adult
hemiplegics these patterns are seen first and may
persist indefinitely. However, in some patients
recovery of normal fractionated movement occurs.
Brunnstrom felt that normal fractionated movement would not be recovered unless the patient
had first gone through the stage of abnormality.
Observations suggest that this may not be true
(Bobath, 1990); during the stage of spinal shock it
may be possible to influence the course of recovery
so that spasticity does not occur or is less severe.
However, even if the patient does have to go
through this stage it would not seem desirable to
augment it.

9.4.3 Reinforcement over time

The Doman-Delacato method for treating brain-
injured children (Tannock, 1976) also developed
from Fay's idea of using abnormal reflex activity.
This method advocates the use of 'patterning'
whereby abnormal activity is encouraged and various forms of sensory stimulation are used to produce it. The sensory stimulation is indiscriminate
and again abnormal movement is being reinforced.
The method advocates the reinforcement of the
effects of treatment through the administration of
intense sensory stimulation and patterned passive
movements for many hours a day by relatives and
their friends. In this respect the method recognized
the need for reinforcement over many hours a day,
something which was not acknowledged by other
approaches.

Conductive education, originally developed in
Hungary in the 1940s by Peto (see Kinsman, 1989;
Todd, 1990), also emphasizes the need for
reinforcement over a long period of time in order
for learning to take place. Treatment techniques
are based on theories of learning and are aimed
at the achievement of functional goals through a
learning of the component subtasks. The main
element used to reinforce performance and achieve
learning is language, whereby patients are taught
to verbalize a task while performing it but other
elements such as continual practice are also used.
Learning of the functional activities and their component subtasks is achieved through reinforcement
by 'conductors' for 24 h a day. In Hungary, children who are educated by this method received
their education while resident in an institution and
there is total commitment to their education by all
concerned. Where the method has been introduced
in the UK, the 24 h commitment has not been
present although centres are now opening which
will attempt to mimic the situation in Hungary.
When the method was used in the rehabilitation of
stroke patients (Kinsman, 1989) it has not been on
a 24 h basis but the other elements of the approach
have been emphasized. These include the setting
of functional goals and the analysis of the function
or task so that the sequence of movements of subtasks can be learned through practice (albeit for a
shorter time per day) and through reinforcement
by language. Provided that the sequences of movements that are reinforced are normal then the
reinforcement for long periods of time should be
more effective than short periods of treatment per
day. However, conductive education does not
involve a physical intervention and therefore no use
is made of the effect of manipulating peripheral
input to change or reinforce output. The method
claims to be effective and to enable children to
achieve a greater potential than they would do
otherwise. A recent study into the use of the
approach in the rehabilitation of stroke patients by
Howard and Verrier (1989) suggested that some
learning of component subtasks took place when
they were reinforced during daily sessions of 1 h
only for 9 months. However, no details of the normality of the movements used for the subtasks are
given and the main criticism of the Peto approach

is that it may lead to the reinforcement of abnormal movement.

9.4.4   The use of artificial electrical stimulation

In the rehabilitation of the muscular system, electrical stimulation has been used to mimic activity in motor nerves and therefore replace the need for active exercise. If electrical stimulation of the same frequency and pattern as the motor unit action potential is applied then this not only causes the muscle to contract but over a period of time it causes long-term functional changes suggested as being due to plastic adaptation (see Chapter 7, Section 7.9 and Kidd *et al.*, 1989). To produce the changes described in Chapter 7, the electrical stimulation was applied for 3 h each day for 10 weeks.

Electrical stimulation has also been used in attempts to modify CNS activity. It has been suggested that high-frequency electrical stimulation of the spinal cord (Sharkey *et al.*, 1982) and the internal capsule (Cooper *et al.*, 1980) can reduce spasticity. Also stimulation of the peripheral nerve to antagonist muscles is suggested as reducing spasticity in the agonists through reciprocal inhibition (Waters *et al.*, 1975). Most studies used a high-frequency stimulation for a short period of time. Reduction of spasticity was reported for up to 3 h in some cases but measurements were mostly of a clinical nature and there were no controls. Bajd *et al.* (1985) used a stimulus frequency of 100 Hz to stimulate the agonists, the spastic quadriceps, by placing the electrodes over the L3 and L4 dermatomes in spinal cord-injured patients. The electrical stimulation did not cause muscle contraction and it was applied for 20 min. The effect on spasticity was measured using the pendulum test (Wartenburg, 1951) and a reduction was found in three out of six patients. However, there was no long-term effect. Shindo and Jones (1987) used an electrical stimulation of a lower frequency (30–40 Hz) over a longer period of time. They stimulated patients with spasticity for a period of six weeks for 9 to 35 min per day. The stimulation was suggested as mimicking manual techniques and was applied to the flexors and extensors cf the knee alternately. Shindo and Jones reported that 30 of 32 patients stimulated had relief of spasticity for 2 to 6 h after the first week of treatment. After the full six weeks of treatment all patients had experienced some relief and 30 for periods up to 78 h. Functionally some patients were said to have a long-term relief that enabled them to walk without any aids. However, measurement of spasticity was by a subjective assessment of activities of daily living and by testing passive joint range (details not given). Again there are no controls.

Electrical stimulation may be one answer to the time element needed if plastic adaptation is to take place in the CNS but if it is to have the required effect of reinforcing normal synaptic chains and normal movement then it must mimic closely the manual techniques that would appear to be effective in the short-term. Also in order to encourage plastic change the stimulation must be of the correct frequency and pattern.

9.4.5   Summary and conclusions

Many different approaches are used in the treatment and rehabilitation of brain-injured patients. Some emphasize the importance of normal movement, others suggest that the presence of abnormal movement can be of use.

The approaches that emphasize normal movement all make use of functional activities or sequences of movement seen in functional activity and all stress the importance of carry-over. Only conductive education, highlighting possible learning difficulties in brain-damaged patients and using learning techniques to try and overcome them, makes use of all 24 h in a day to ensure maximum carry-over. However, this approach does not use physical intervention to attempt to achieve normality.

Some approaches make use of abnormal reflex activity and suggest that it should be used as a path to normality. One of these approaches emphasizes the reinforcement of the abnormal activity for up to 16 h per day.

Artificial electrical stimulation has been used in the treatment of brain-injured patients, particularly those with spasticity. So far the approach has not combined the production of normal activity or sequences of movement with that of stress of the CNS with the correct trophic code over a long period of time each day.

9.5   A guide to effective therapeutic intervention

Effective therapeutic intervention needs to emphasize the following:

1. *The facilitation of normal movement*

An effective therapy must facilitate normal movement through natural means (i.e. handling) or through artificial stimulation. Normal movement will facilitate normal movement. This should strengthen and maintain muscles for functional tasks. It should also, in the case of spasticity, lead to a prevention of length-associated changes and reduce the spasticity through the opening of pathways for normal movement. Normal movement should also include normal automatic postural adjustments and through their use should preserve these. Therefore normal movement should include:

(a) Automatic postural adjustments occurring both during and before the movement.
(b) Normal patterns of voluntary movement in distal limbs to achieve specific functions or goals.

Normal movement can be facilitated through the use of appropriate afferent input from the periphery as indicated by studies into the neural control of movement. If artificial stimulation is to be used then it must be a stimulation of muscles in a correct sequence for normal movement and must contain the trophic code.

2. *The need to stress the central nervous system over a period of time in order to reinforce plastic adaptation to normal movement*

If plastic adaptation is to occur in the CNS then the system needs to be stressed. Axonal sprouting begins immediately within the spinal cord following CNS damage because there is no other guiding force other than the attraction exerted by denuded synapses. When plastic adaptation has been shown to occur within muscles, it has been caused by an electrical stimulation which is applied for several hours per day. Between stimulations the muscle will usually be resting. Any activity however would only lead to a reinforcing of the stimulus effect. If stimulation is to be applied to the CNS in patients with lesions to the brain or spinal cord then it would need to be for at least a comparable time with no other adverse stimuli occurring in between. Unfortunately patients with CNS damage do move and they do so abnormally. If a stimulus for normal movement is applied even for several hours in a day, either artificially or by handling, the patient may provide his own abnormal stimulus for the rest of the time. This abnormal stimulus would be the most stressing and would therefore be the one to effect changes.

Therefore, for normal movement and handling to be used to facilitate normal movement there must be a carry-over effect if plastic change is to occur. Techniques recommended to reinforce learning should be of help when used alongside techniques used to facilitate normal movement.

If artificial stimulation is to be used to facilitate normal movement then it must be given for long enough to make it the overriding effect on the CNS. More research is needed to identify the correct sequence and pattern of stimulation needed and also the correct sites for stimulation.

This book has presented a picture of a nervous system that is able to adapt to changes forced upon it during development and during recovery from disease or injury. This nervous system is sufficiently complex to be able to control human behaviour but sufficiently flexible to be able to restore human behaviour once it has been impaired. This restoration is achieved by the nervous system adapting to a changing environment. In physical rehabilitation this adaptation could lead to abnormal movement but if guided the adaptation could be to a normal pattern of activity. The ideas presented in this book lead to the adoption of a particular approach to therapeutic intervention; one aimed at achieving normal movement and reinforcing that normality. In this way it is felt that patients may achieve their full potential following brain damage.

References

Ashburn, A. (1982) A physical assessment of stroke patients. *Physiotherapy* **68**: 109–13.

Ashby, P. and Verrier, M. (1980) Human motoneurone responses to group I volleys blocked presynaptically by vibration. *Brain Research* **184**: 511-16.

Ashby, P., Verrier, M., Carleton, S. and Somerville, J. (1980) Vibratory inhibition of the monosynaptic reflex and presynaptic inhibition in man. In Feldman, R. G., Young, R. R. and Koella, W. P., eds. *Spasticity: Disordered Motor Control.* Chicago: Year Book Medical Publications, pp. 335–44.

Bajd, T., Gregoric, M., Vodovnik, L. and Benko, H. (1985) Electrical stimulation in treating spasticity resulting from spinal cord injury. *Archives of Physical Medicine and Rehabilitation* **66**: 515–17.

Bobath, B. (1963) Treatment principles and planning in cerebral palsy. *Physiotherapy* **49**: 122–4.

Bobath, B. (1971) *Abnormal Postural Reflex Activity Caused by Brain Lesions.* London: Heinemann.

Bobath, B. (1990) *Adult Hemiplegia: Evaluation and Treatment.* 3rd edition. London: Heinemann.

Brunnstrom, S. (1961) Motor behaviour of adult hemiplegic patients. *American Journal of Occupational Therapy* **15**: 6–12.

Brunnstrom, S. (1970) *Movement Therapy in Hemiplegia*. New York: Harper and Row.

Burke, D. (1980) A reassessment of the muscle spindle contribution to muscle tone in normal and spastic man. In Feldman, R. G., Young, R. R. and Koella, W. P., eds. *Spasticity: Disordered Motor Control*. Chicago: Year Book Medical Publications, pp. 261–78.

Burke, D. (1988) Spasticity as an adaptation to pyramidal tract injury. In Waxman, S. G., ed. *Advances in Neurology*. Volume 47. *Functional Recovery in Neurological Disease*. New York: Raven Press, pp. 401–23.

Burke, D. and Lance, J. W. (1973) Studies of the reflex effects of primary and secondary spindle endings in spasticity. In Desmedt, J. E., ed. *New Developments in EMG and Clinical Neurophysiology*. Volume 3. Basel: Karger, pp. 475–95.

Burke, D., Hagbarth, K. E., Lofstedt, L. and Wallin, B. G. (1976) The response of human muscle spindle endings to vibration during isometric contractions. *Journal of Physiology* **261**: 695–711.

Carr, J. H. and Shepherd, R. B. (1989) A motor learning model for stroke rehabilitation. *Physiotherapy* **75**: 372–80.

Cook, T. and Cozzens, B. (1976) Human solutions for locomotion: III. The initiation of gait. In Herman, R. M., Grillner, S., Stein, P. S. G. and Stuart, D. G., eds. *Neural Control of Locomotion*. New York: Plenum Publishing Corporation, pp. 65–77.

Cooper, I. S., Upton, A. R. M. and Amin, I. (1980) Reversibility of chronic neurologic deficits: Some effects of elctrical stimulation of the thalamus and the internal capsule in man. *Applied Neurophysiology* **43**: 244–58.

Devor, M., Merrill, E. G. and Wall, P. D. (1977) Dorsal horn cells that respond to stimulation of distant dorsal roots. *Journal of Physiology* **270**: 519–31.

Dindar, F. and Verrier, M. (1975) Studies on the receptor responsible for vibration induced inhibition of monosynaptic reflexes in man. *Journal of Neurology, Neurosurgery and Psychiatry* **38**: 155–60.

Eccles, E. and Lundberg, A. (1958) Integrative patterns of Ia synaptic actions on motorneurones of hip and knee muscles. *Journal of Physiology* **144**: 271–98.

Eldred, E. and Hagbarth, K-E. (1954) Facilitation and inhibition of gamma efferents by stimulation of certain skin areas. *Journal of Neurophysiology* **17**: 59–65.

Eklund, G. and Hagbarth, K. E. (1966) Normal variabilility of tonic vibration reflexes in man. *Experimental Neurology* **16**: 80–92.

Fay, T. (1948) The neurophysical aspects of therapy in cerebral palsy. *Archives of Physical Medicine* **29**: 327–34.

Fay, T. (1954) Basic considerations regarding neuromuscular and reflex therapy. *Spastics Quarterly* **3**: 5–8.

Forget, R., Hultborn, H., Meunier, S., Pantieri, R. and Pierrot-Deseilligny, E. (1989) Facilitation of quadriceps motorneurones by group I afferents from pretibial flexors in man. 2. Changes occurring during voluntary contractions. *Experimental Brain Research* **78**: 21–7.

Forssberg, H., Grillner, S. and Rossignol, S. (1975) Phase dependent reflex reversal during walking in chronic spinal cats. *Brain Research* **85**: 103–7.

Gillies, J. D., Lance, J. W., Neilson, P. D. and Tassinari, C. A. (1969) Presynaptic inhibition of the monosynaptic reflex. *Journal of Physiology* **205**: 329–39.

Goldberger, M. E. and Murray, M. (1988) Patterns of sprouting and implications for recovery of function. In Waxman, S. G., ed. *Advances in Neurology*. Volume 47. *Functional Recovery in Neurological Disease*. New York: Raven Press.

Grillner, S. (1981) Control of locomotion in bipedes, tetrapodes and fish. In Brooks, V., ed. *Handbook of Physiology*. Volume III, Section I. *The Nervous System II. Motor Control*. American Physiological Society. Baltimore: Waverley Press, pp. 1179–1236.

Grillner, S. and Rossignol, S. (1978) Contralateral reflex reversal controlled by limb position in the acute spinal cat injected with clonidine i.v. *Brain Research* **144**: 411-4.

Herman, R., Cook, T., Cozzens, B. and Freedman, W. (1973) Control of postural reactions in man: the initiation of gait. In Stein, R. B., Pearson, K. G., Smith, R. S. and Redford, J. B., eds. *Control of Posture and Locomotion*. New York: Plenum Publishing Corporation, pp. 363–88.

Howard, R. and Verrier, M. (1989) Conductive education approach for retraining motor performance in patients with long-standing hemiparesis: case studies. *Physiotherapy Canada* **41**: 204–8.

Kabat, H. (1952) Studies on neuromuscular dysfunction: XV. The role of central facilitation in restoration of motor function in paralysis. *Archives of Physical Medicine* **33**: 521–33.

Kidd, G. L., Oldham, J. A. and Stanley, J. K. (1989) Eutrophic electrotherapy and atrophied muscles: a pilot clinical trial. *Clinical Rehabilitation* **2**: 219–30.

Kinsman, R. (1989) A conductive education approach to stroke patients at Barnet General Hospital. *Physiotherapy* **75**: 418–21.

Knott, M. and Voss, D. (1969) Proprioceptive neuromuscular facilitation. New York: Harper and Row.

Lundberg, A. (1979) Multisensory control of spinal reflex pathways. *Progress in Brain Research* **50**: 11–28.

Maehlen, J. and Arid, N. (1982) The effects of electrical stimulation on sprouting after partial denervation of guinea pig sympathetic ganglion cells. *Journal of Physiology* **322**: 151–66.

Magnus, R. (1909) Regelung der bewegungen durch das zentralnervensystem. Mitteilung I. *Pflugers Archiv für die Gesamte Physiologie des Menschen und der Tiere* **130**: 219–52.

Magnus, R. (1926) Some results of studies in the physiology of posture. *Lancet* **ii**: 531–6, 585–8.

McLellan, D. L. and Hassan, N. H. (1982) The use of EMGs to assess impaired voluntary movement associated with increased muscle tone. *Electroencephalography and Clinical Neurophysiology* **36**: 169–71 (Supplement).

Miller, S. and Musa, I. M. (1982) The significance of hip movement and vertical loading on the foot in the evaluation and retraining of gait in stroke patients. *Proceedings of the IXth WCPT International Congress*, pp. 765–71.

Nance, P. W., Shears, A. H. and Nance, D. M. (1989) Reflex changes induced by clonidine in spinal cord injured patients. *Paraplegia* **27**: 296–301.

Neilson, P. D. (1972) Interaction between voluntary contraction and tonic strength reflex transmission in normal and spastic patients. *Journal of Neurology, Neurosurgery and Psychiatry* **35**: 853–60.

Perry, J. (1969) The mechanics of walking in hemiplegia. *Clinical Orthopaedics and Related Research* **63**: 23–31.

Pierrot-Deseilligny, E., Bergego, C., Katz, R. *et al*. (1981a) Cutaneous depression of Ib reflex pathways to motorneurones in man. *Experimental Brain Research* **42**: 351–61.

Pierrot-Deseilligny, E., Morin, C., Bergego, C. and Tankov, N. (1981b) Pattern of group I fibre projections from ankle flexor and extensor muscles in man. *Experimental Brain Research* **42**: 337–50.

Rood, M. (1956) Neurophysiological mechanisms utilized in the treatment of neuromuscular dysfunction. *American Journal of Occupational Therapy* **10**: 220–5.

Rossignol, S. and Gautier, L. (1980) Reversal of contralateral limb reflexes. *Proceedings of the International Union of the Physiological Sciences* **13**: 639.

Sharkey, P. C., Dimitrijevic, M. M. and Faganel, J. (1982) Neurophysiological analysis of factors influencing efficacy of spinal cord stimulation. *Applied Neurophysiology* **45**: 68–72.

Sheikh, K., Smith, D. S., Meade, T. W. and Brennan, P. J. (1978) Methods and problems of a stroke rehabilitation trial. *British Journal of Occupational Therapy* **41**: 262–5.

Shindo, N. and Jones, R. (1987) Reciprocal patterned electrical stimulation of the lower limbs in severe spasticity. *Physiotherapy* **73**: 579–82.

Tannock, R. (1976) Doman-Delacato method for treating brain-injured children: an assessment. *Physiotherapy Canada* **28**: 203–9.

Todd, J. E. (1990) Conductive education: the continuing challenge. *Physiotherapy* **76**: 13–16.

Uexkull, J. von (1904) Die ersten ursachen des rhythmus in der tierreihe. *Ergebnisse Physiologie* **3**: 1–11.

Wall, P. D. (1980) Mechanisms of plasticity of connection following damage in adult mammalian nervous systems. In Bach-y-Rita, P., ed. *Recovery of Function: Theoretical Considerations for Brain Injury Rehabilitation*. Baltimore: University Park Press, pp. 91–105.

Wall, P. D. and Werman, R. (1976) Physiology and anatomy of long ranging afferent fibres within the spinal cord. *Journal of Physiology* **255**: 321–34.

Wartenburg, R. (1951) Pendulousness of legs as diagnostic test. *Neurology* **1**: 18–24.

Waters, R., McNeal, D. and Perry, J. (1975) Experimental correction of footdrop by electrical stimulation of the peroneal nerve. *Journal of Bone and Joint Surgery (American)* **57**: 1047–54.

Appendix

1. The sentence quoted below is taken from Section 3.1 in Chapter 3 and it summarizes both points in the Appendix to this book.

It is difficult to see how molecules, which we comprehend as 'chemistry', can be so effective in generating electric potential and current flow, which we comprehend, with equivalent determination, as 'physics'.

Figure A.1 was introduced first as Fig. 3.2 in Chapter 3. Since then the subject had been presented to you in a way that should make the rock-hard definitions 'chemistry' and 'physics' appear simplistic. At the fringe, where living meets non-living, a totally new science appears. Without it, neither the developing neuroscience nor the attainable rehabilitation would be realized.

The components of the circuit diagram shown as Fig. A.1 are not electronic, they operate by inducing and modifying the flow of ions. We have mentioned already that the capacitor C_m shown to the right of Fig. A.1a holds the electric charge as does any other capacitor in an electronic device, but it is composed not of metal foil and waxed paper insulators but consists of the resistive elements of the neuron membrane (the lipids) and the conducting sheets of the electrolyte solutions on either side.

The membrane capacitor slows down the development of a changing membrane potential as the neuron responds to a stimulus. This is an explanation of the basis of the 'strength duration curve' that is still a valid measure of excitability in the clinical context.

The conductance elements represent 'the ease with which different ions flow into and out of the neuron', for that reason it is referred to sometimes as a 'gate'. One might prefer the image of sheep, but it is ions that we are stuck with. The ion pump works as an electrogenic pump and operates in an antiport manner, moving sodium and potassium ions in different directions. The ease with which ions flow is determined by ionophores, which themselves are sensitive to the potential difference across the membrane, which is of course of molecular dimensions. A remarkably sensitive feedback exists therefore between the ionophore which allows the potential difference to change as ions permitted to flow by the ionophore exert their electrical effect. Do not forget that each ion flowing carries with it an electric charge. So,

in simple terms, what allows ions to flow is themselves controlled by the consequence of that flow.

Adding to the excitement a little, suppose we play Fig. A.2 with the other hand. It illustrates the propagation and transmissions of electrical signals (action potentials) over a simple axon (a) and over a simple axon where electrical continuity is interrupted by a septum (b). This sort of electrical synapse is found in primitive nervous systems, and occasionally in ours. It is with example (c) that we are introduced to the improbability of synaptic transmission. Not only that, we should now take on board the idea of the improbability of a synapse. The symbols are for the perfectionist, but we feel that the nub of the whole argument is that the improbability of a synapse is a controlled improbability. As a rehabilitation specialist you should now be feeling the surge of achievement as you realize that you can both understand and employ the controls of improbability by directing the placement of appropriate molecules in the membranes implied by Fig. A.2. You do not have to place them in the membranes in the literal sense: change the environment of the neuromuscular system, and the nuclei will work themselves to the bone in instructing the neuron to undertake the synthesis of molecules appropriate for the task.

Is that time here again when the need for a darkened room and a dampened cloth looms large? Fear not: Fig. A.3 is an ideal anodyne for the pain: you were never promised that the subject at this intensity would not hurt your head! Figure A.3 introduces diagrammatically the idea that a pressure can be created across the neuron membrane. In fact, the development of two pressures is attempted. One of them for Na^+ and the other for K^+. Think first in terms of pressure expressed as concentration difference across the neuron membrane. Long ago, when we were innocent we introduced the concept of intracellular and extracellular fluid compartments.

K^+ High concentration	K^+ Low concentration
INSIDE	OUTSIDE
Na^+ Low concentration	Na^+ High concentration

Firstly, the pressure due to Na^+ and K^+ is represented by the height of the two columns drawn on both sides of the membrane. At this stage of things everything is at

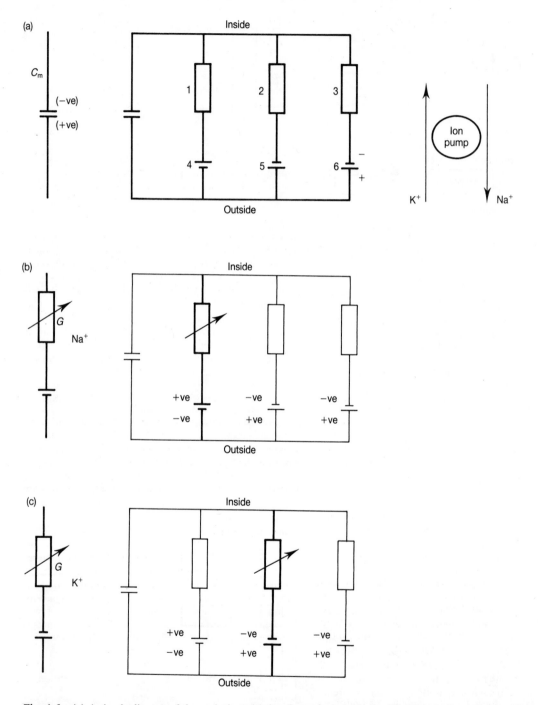

Fig. A.1 (a) A simple diagram of the equivalent circuits of a neuron membrane. The electrical capacitance (C_m) keeps apart and holds the electric charge that is formed across it (polarization). An ion pump linked to the neuron metabolism is able to move Na^+ and K^+ in opposite directions and is able also to transport them against their concentration gradients. Circuit elements 4 and 5 are ion pumps for Na^+ and K^+, respectively. Element 6 is the electric potential which is able to direct leakage outflow of ions of −ve electric charge (e.g. Cl^-). (b) and (c) Rectangles 1, 2 and 3 are ion specific channels which allow ion conductivity changes (G_{Na+} and G_K^+) as a signal of an excitatory response by the neuron.

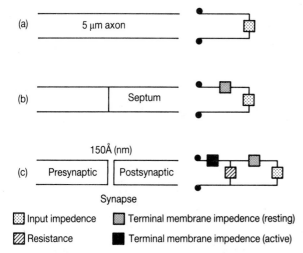

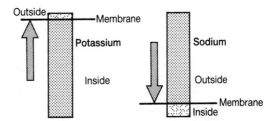

Fig. A.3 Concentration pressures and electrical pressures. The K^+ and Na^+ exert a concentration pressure from inside to outside (K^+) and outside to inside (Na^+). The net unstimulated electrical pressure or potential operates in the opposite direction.

Fig. A.2 Cable characteristics of an axon can be applied only to the most simple situations. (a) A small diameter non-myelinated axon adds only an impedence characteristic to transmission. (b) Should the continuity of the cable be interrupted by a septum a second element of impedence is introduced. (c) When a synaptic cleft is also introduced, the number of both resistive and impedence elements is increased. This argues that when transmission is compared with propagation, something other than electrical, cable transmission must be introduced. This is the presynaptic release of transmitter molecules and the reaction of them with molecular receptors in the postsynaptic membrane. Definitions: Full definition of terms, which could be unfamiliar to you, will be found in the Glossary.

the difficulty of plumbing. Potassium bits would try to escape from the inside, and sodium bits would attempt to flood in. But the bits carry a positive electric charge: they are ions. To concentration pressure we must add, therefore, an electrical pressure. The difference in pressure is maintained by the electrogenic pumps acting as antiports. The arrows with horizontal shading represent both pressures applied to the membrane. So the bits, the dots of Fig. A.3, attempt to carry electric charges, which, when associated with the bits, cancel carefully the two opposing tendencies: until that is a stimulus operates channels for the ions and unbalances the entire system. The facts of life have made themselves known. Modify the molecules at the heart of all this and you modify the activity of the neuromuscular system. Which is exactly what this book is all about!

2. To open the second part of this appendix suppose we examine one of the simpler bits of chemistry introduced in the book. Figure A.4 will expose the trickery of biochemistry and render clear the obscurity. Now where did I read ESCHEW OBFUSCATION? ATP is one of the key molecules in living systems. This figure appeared

first as Fig. 1.10. It has been suggested that a rocket with a pay load of fire-fly tails should be despatched to Mars. If, when it arrived there, a glow could be seen from earth by optical telescope the existence of life on the planet would be proven. The chemical affinity of fire-fly tails for ATP is legendary. If:

$$\text{Fire-fly tails} + \text{Mars} = \text{Luminescence}$$
$$\text{Fire-fly tails} + \text{ATP} = \text{Luminescence}$$
$$ergo$$
$$\text{there is ATP on Mars}$$
$$ergo$$
$$\text{there is life on Mars}$$

We can ignore much of the detail of chemistry and focus our minds on the 'strain' built up in the molecule by the linking together of the five molecules. It will suffice to say that the 'strain' appears to be concentrated to the last two of the three phosphate groups: the tail of the molecule. The energy of the two bonds is modest by

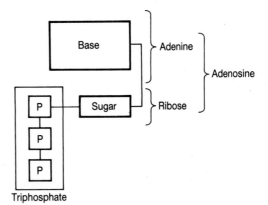

Fig. A.4 Another diagrammatic representation dissects the adenosine triphosphate (ATP) molecule. An organic base (adenine) is combined with a five-carbon sugar (a pentose called ribose) which carries three phosphate groups.

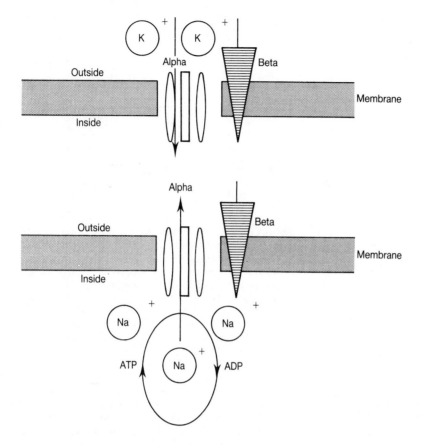

Fig. A.5 A diagrammatic illustration of a membrane macromolecule acting as an ion pump. The alpha-unit of the protein acts as an ATPase. The beta-unit, a glycoprotein, is incompletely understood. Conformational changes of the alpha-unit of the protein acts as a contrapump moving Na^+ and K^+ ions across the membrane against their respective concentration gradients. In the two diagrams of Fig. 3.4, the pumping actions are shown as being separate. They are in fact one. This presentation is to ease understanding. Refer once again to the text of Chapter 3 and to Chapter 1, Section 1.1.

comparison with many bond energies in biochemistry (Table A.1).

What is 'high' is the amount of that energy in that particular bond – when it can be applied to another

Table A.1

Reaction	Free energies of hydrolysis kcal mole $^{-1}$
Phosphoenylpyruvate to pyruvate + P_i	−13.0
Phosphocreatine to creatine + P_i	−10.3
ATP to ADP+Pi	**−8.0**
Acetylcoenzyme A to acetate + CoA	−7.5
Polypeptide$n$ to 2 polypeptide$_{n/2}$	−0.5

The free energy available when the reactions described go to completion in 1000 calories per molecular weight in grams.

These figures have been selected from Dyson, R. D. (1974) *Cell Biology: A Molecular Approach*. Boston: Allyn and Bacon.

chemical reaction. The writer lectures to undergraduates in physical education. They worship at the shrine of the high energy bond. When I tell them that I do not have two high energy bonds to rub together, they are not impressed by that either.

The molecule is accessible to the enzyme ATPase and, you have guessed it, the electrogenic ion pump itself is an ATPase. Figure A.5, which was introduced as Fig. 3.3, shows, in diagram, how the applicable energy of ATP can be applied, through the agency of ATPase, to the complex protein (with its alpha and beta components) which acts simultaneously on Na^+ and K^+, in antiport fashion, to transform the applicable bond energy into an electrical potential difference.

Was it not the Players in Hamlet who performed a Comical, Historical Tragedy; or could it have been a Tragical, Comical History? It is only a matter of time before you talk learnedly about biochemical physics and physical biochemistry, and those without the blessed light of reason will be under the opinion that you are discussing two separate subjects. But we know differently. You are on the brink of life itself: come on in, the water is lovely.

Glossary

Key: cf. = compare and contrast with. q.v. = the reference will give further information and add to your understanding.

We acknowledge the usefulness of Abercrombie, Hickman and Johnson (1973) and Reber (1985) without whose writing, fundamental accuracy would have been totally lacking.

actin   the protein *monomer* (q.v.) from which microfilaments are made. It is involved in cell movement, cell shape and the guidance of the *growth cone* (q.v.).

actin   a protein component of a neuron membrane. Found as nodal points in *mechanoceptors* (q.v.).

actin   of skeletal muscle. A complex of protein molecules that is involved with myosin in the mechanical action of the *myofilament* (q.v.). The complex is formed of tropomyosin and the actin monomers.

action or **active**   a loose way of saying excited (q.v.) resting.

action potential   changes in the potential difference across a cell membrane, particularly neuronal including some dendritic and muscular membranes, caused by the opening of *ionophores* (q.v.). The interior of the cell always becomes less negative. It is described for any one cell as being 'all-or-nothing' (q.v.).

adaptation   to a particular activity, of a cell or tissue, refers to a character which makes possible, or improves, performance of that activity.

adenine   an organic base (q.v.). A component of DNA. A component of the molecules AMP, ADP and ATP (q.v.).

adenylate cyclase   an enzyme that converts adenosine triphosphate (ATP) to cyclic adenosine monophosphate cAMP (q.v.).

ADP   adenosine diphosphate. A family of molecules with a general structure of *base + sugar + phosphate*. Coenzymes operating to transfer bond energy to cooperating molecules in metabolic reactions.

adrenergic   a definition which emphasizes the name of the molecule that is effective in bringing about an action such as synaptic transmission. The suffix -ergic refers to the effect, q.v. cholinergic.

'all-or-nothing'   a description of the characteristics of an action potential. What is meant is that the amplitude of an action potential is a factor of the cell membrane and, when developed, not of the stimulus intensity. There is no such thing as a large and a small action potential in the same cell.

allosteric   translates as 'another form'. Allosteric changes take place, for example, when a membrane molecule changes form and in so doing 'pumps' an ion uphill or against a concentration gradient.

AMP   adenosine monophosphate is associated with similar bases, thymine, cytosine guanine and uracil (q.v.). With the phosphate group attached at both ends (3′–5′) it adopts a cyclic form (cyclic AMP) and operates in the cell as a second messenger (q.v.).

amu (**a**tomic **m**ass **u**nit)   the weight (or more exactly the mass) of the hydrogen atom (1/16 of the weight of the oxygen atom). A unit for expressing the weight of a macromolecule. Sometimes referred to as a 'dalton'.

anticodon   a three nucleotide sequence in a chromosome or mRNA chain which complements the *codon* (q.v.) in information transfer during the synthesis of a polypeptide chain.

antiport   translates as carrying different ions across a cell membrane simultaneously but in opposite directions. Refers, in the context of this book, to macromolecules of the neuron membrane acting as *electrogenic* ion pumps.

APUD   an acronym for 'amine precursor uptake and decarboxylation' system. It is believed to derive embryologically from a common type of neuroectodermal precursor cell. An important stage in thinking which refused to separate endocrine and nervous activities q.v. gut/brain hormones.

association fibres   cerebral cortical axons linking cortical regions in the same hemisphere.

associative learning   the learning whereby one stimulus implies another.

astrocytes   glial cells with several processes, giving them a star-shaped appearance.

ATP   adenosine triphosphate. With a phosphate group at the 3′ position, the molecule behaves as a 'high energy' bond donor.

atrophy   the state of being deprived of a trophic influence: e.g. nutrient, agent or contact with nerve or nervous discharge exerting a trophic (q.v.) effect.

autoproteolysis   literally, self-digesting or more specifically a cell system which breaks down or digests its own protein molecules.

axon hillock   the location on the soma (cell body) of a neuron where an action potential is generated to be propagated over the rest of the neuronal surface.

axonal sprouting   the growth of new branches from an axon into a region that it did not previously innervate.

axonal transport   an intracellular mechanism by which neuronal components, either subcellular structures or macromolecules, are carried. The transport may be anterograde or orthograde (cell body to periphery) or retrograde (periphery to cell body). A form of information transmission by neurons other than by action potential.

base (organic)   a molecule owing its basic character to an oxygen or a nitrogen atom. A molecule possessing a lone pair of electrons used in the formation of a coordinate bond. Examples of organic bases are adenine and guanine (q.v.).

biophysics   a subdivision of biology which treats phenomena in the terms of physics. An example is the quantification of the membrane potential and the ways in which it changes as a system moves, in both directions, between the states of inactivity and activity.

birthday   the day on which a cell is produced by the final division of its parent cell.

booster   jargon for an active patch of molecules in a neuron membrane. These 'boost' the decaying electrotonic currents by regenerating the action potential which initiated the whole process. See saltatory (q.v.) conduction.

cable characteristics   are described to simplify the concepts of transmission of electrical signals in nerve and muscle. The cable characteristics of a neuron allow the conduction of electronic currents and explain the saltatory (q.v.) propagation once an action potential is generated in a myelinated axon.

calmodulin   a protein that can bind Ca^{2+}, after which it activates a number of intracellular processes.

capacitance   an electrical system of conductors separated by insulators able to store an electric charge when an electrical potential difference exists between the conductors. The bilayer of the cell membrane represents a capacitance which stores the electric charge established by ion pumps, and the passive redistribution of ions which occurs due to the electric charge. The special membrane molecules responsible for the charge are called the electrogenic pumps (q.v.) and are comprised of special protein molecules able to act as ion pumps (cf.) antiports.

cathode   a negative electrode attracting positive ions.

cholinergic   releasing acetylcholine as effector molecule.

cistron   a gene defined functionally as a length of DNA producing the RNA molecules which in turn produce

a specific polypeptide chain to function in cellular activity.

CMOS   acronym for a form of silicon chip composed of a **C**ompatible **M**etallic **O**xide and **S**ilicon which has very low electrical power consumption and so spares the batteries of portable devices.

codon   a unit in the genetic code. Consisting of three adjacent bases of nucleotide molecules arranged along a chromosome or tRNA chain. The three successive bases guanine-adenine-cytosine (G-A-C) for example is the codon for the incorporation of the amino acid alanine into the polypeptide being assembled.

commissural fibres   cerebral cortical axons linking one hemisphere to the other.

corpus striatum   the caudate, putamen and globus pallidus. A major component of the basal ganglia.

cortex, motorsensory (**Ms**)   in today's neurology there is a move away from the Brodmann classification of the cerebral cortex into such areas as 4, 6 and 3-1-2. Areas of the cerebral cortex previously thought of as motor in function contribute to sensory perception. Similarly, an area once thought of as serving sensation is recognized now as contributing to motor control. A similar change in definition recognizes a dominantly sensory cortex with some motor capability. (abbv. **Sm**).

cortical plate   the layer in the developing forebrain into which neurons migrate to form eventually the adult cortical grey matter.

cytotactin   cell-substrate adhesion molecule found on glial cells. Its adhesive properties depend on extracellular calcium ion.

dendritic potentials   changes of variable amplitude in the potential difference across a dendritic membrane, caused by the binding of a transmitter molecule to a ligand (q.v.) operated ionophore (q.v.). Unlike the change caused by action potentials, the inside of the cell can become more negative or more positive (q.v.) hot-spot.

depolarization   a membrane event leading to a change in membrane potential. When the change reaches threshold for the membrane, there is a transition from depolarization to reverse polarization of the membrane and the development of an action potential.

depolarization   (of axon terminals) is associated with the release of neurotransmitter (q.v.) molecules. The depolarization here leads to the development of a postsynaptic potential (PSP) across the membrane of the cell on the other side of the synapse or endplate. Postsynaptic potentials can give rise to inhibitory postsynaptic potentials (IPSPs) as well as excitatory postsynaptic potentials (EPSPs).

depolymerize   remove monomers from a polymer (q.v.).

diacyl glycerol   a combination of two chains of fatty acids linked to glycerol. Released from phosphatydyl inositol biphosphate, diacyl glycerol helps to activate protein kinase C. It is important in cell signalling.

diploid the state of a cell nucleus when it has a full complement of chromosomes, so that twice the haploid (q.v.) number is present. In humans the diploid number is 46.

dipole the separation of unlike electric charges within the same molecule. With the appropriate charge (either +ve or −ve) orienting the dipole towards the charge on an ion (q.v.). The ion and the surrounding water molecules determine the size of the hydrated ion and hence its passage through membranes. See hydrosphere.

dopaminergic a neuron which exerts its effect by releasing dopamine.

endocytosis the internalization of a part of the cell membrane by pinching it off to form an intracellular vesicle.

electrogenic the contribution to the membrane potential of ion pumps acting as antiports (q.v.) and establishing an asymmetric distribution of ions across the membrane.

endocrine a system which signals by means of molecules circulating in blood plasma. The molecules, known as hormones, are important agents of control. cf. paracrine and neurocrine.

endorphins endogenous morphine-like substances that are believed to be neuroactive. A naturally occurring substance behaving as morphine itself does, i.e. being both pain killing and addictive (q.v.) enkephalins.

enkephalin two naturally occurring pentapeptide molecules. They belong to series of similar molecules which are involved in the natural suppression of pain.

fasciculation the association of axons to form bundles.

fibronectin a protein found in the extracellular matrix, capable of binding to cells and to other components of the extracellular matrix.

filopodia thin processes protruding from the growth cone (q.v.). They are crucial to the directional guidance of the growth cone.

fodrin a protein that affects the linkage of cytoskeletal elements to each other and to the cell membrane.

fusimotor fusimotoneurons (once called gamma-), systems of motoneurons and axons which are motor to intra**fusal** (inside the spindle-shaped structure) muscles. Intrafusal muscle fibres are exclusive to the muscle spindle receptor. It is believed that a fusimotor system is represented at all levels of the neuraxis. It regulates the responsiveness of the receptor to static and dynamic phases of stretching.

G-proteins proteins that bind guanidine triphosphate (GTP). Second messengers (q.v.). They are activated by the binding of a ligand (q.v.) to a receptor protein, and in turn they activate or inhibit an enzyme such as adenylate cyclase (q.v.).

GAP a growth-associated protein (q.v.).

GAP43 a particular growth-associated protein playing a fundamental part in development, regeneration and learning. It binds calmodulin (q.v.) and releases it when appropriate.

gene a sequence of nucleic acid bases that code in biosynthesis for a protein.

gene expression the degree to which particular genes or inherited traits are displayed phenotype(ically) (q.v.). Environmental effects, in the sense used in this book, dictate gene expression.

genome all of the genes of a particular species.

genotype genetic constitution of an organism, as contrasted with the characteristics manifested by the organism. The potentiality of the organism. It is possible for cells to have the same genotype but different phenotypes as they respond to environmentally produced adaptations (q.v. phenotype). Genotype = potentiality, but phenotype = actuality.

growth-associated proteins proteins that bind calmodulin (q.v.), releasing it in response to signals inducing growth.

growth cone the expanded tip of a neurite (q.v.) where material is added to an elongating axon or dendrite. It is motile and exploratory. Its membrane is replete with molecules of an informational quality. It is, in the sense of molecular neurobiology, the origin of growth-related signals and a receptor of similar signals.

gut/brain hormones e.g. the molecules cholecystokinin and gastrin are now called neuroactive peptides. They, or molecules which resemble them closely, are believed to play a dual role as neurotransmitter and a controlling hormone on the gastrointestinal tract. Believed to act in the appetite/satiety behavioural system.

H-reflex an abbreviation for Hoffman reflex. A procedure for measuring the excitability of skeletomotoneuron pools. An electric stimulus is applied percutaneously to a peripheral nerve trunk. Calculation from the ratio of the amplitude of the electric discharge of skeletal muscle fibres (their action potentials) excited directly by the stimulus to the motor axons, and the action potentials evoked in the same muscle by the same stimulus, operating over a monosynaptic reflex arc.

habilitation involves the development of an ability, frequently a motor ability, not previously held by an individual.

haploid having a single set of chromosomes in each cell nucleus. The number of chromosomes in each gamete (sex cell). Characteristic of gametes. One half of the diploid number.

'hard-wired' as opposed to plastic. Jargon for a description of a nervous system incapable of undergoing plastic adaptation.

heterophilic liking another. Binding of one kind of molecule to a different kind.

homophilic   liking the same. Binding of one molecule to another of the same kind.

hot spots   on axons and dendrites. The sites of transition from an electronic transmission of the graded and non-propagated changes of excitation to 'all-or-nothing' (q.v.) action potentials that are propagated over the neuronal membrane. Sometimes referring particularly to the axon hillock or to nodes of Ranvier.

hydrosphere   a volume within the body fluid compartments occupied by an electrically charged ion (q.v.) and the 'atmosphere' of electrically charged water molecule dipoles (q.v.) attracted to it. One factor determining the passage of ions through membranes.

inferior colliculus   an elevation on the dorsal aspect of the midbrain, forming a part of the auditory pathway.

impedence   the opposition (resistance) to a changing or alternating current flow.

input impedence   the opposition to a changing or alternating current flow entering an electrical network.

inositol   a sugar found in phosphatidyl inositol biphosphate and inositol triphosphate.

integrins   molecules found in cell membranes, capable of binding to extracellular matrix molecules such as laminin (q.v.).

ionophores   a protein in the cell membrane with a channel that can open or close, under the influence of the potential difference across the membrane, to control the passage of ions.

laminin   a protein found in the extracellular matrix in the basal lamina. It appears during development and regeneration of the nervous system and guides growth cones (q.v.) by binding to integrins (q.v.) in their membranes.

lamellipodium   a thin veil of cell membrane containing actin microfilaments, draped between the filopodia (q.v.) of growth cones (q.v.). Lamellipodia are probably where new membrane is added to a growing neurite (q.v.).

lateral geniculate nucleus   a swelling on the ventral surface of the thalamus. It is a part of the visual pathway linking the retina to the striate cortex.

ligand   molecules that are electron donors. They serve in bonding, binding or tying molecules together.

ligand-gated channels   ion channels that open when a ligand (q.v.) as a neurotransmitter binds to them.

long-term potentiation   the enhanced effectiveness of a synapse resulting from high-frequency stimulation. It lasts for months and possibly very much longer.

lower motoneuron disorder   a disorder characterized by muscle weakness or flaccidity due to damage to the motor cells of the ventral horn of the spinal cord (or of the brain stem nuclei) or their axons. The concept of a lower motoneuron presupposed the existence of an upper motoneuron whose cell body and axon lies above the lower motoneuron and entirely within the CNS. Any lesion of the upper motoneuron was thought once to result in spasticity. The concept of an upper motoneuron has been superceded by the idea of many groups of axons, all with differing functions, descending from the brain to the spinal cord. Some descending groups of axons may suffer lesion without resulting in a spastic paralysis.

lysosomes   intracellular bags (vesicles) of enzymes that break down molecules. They are the refuse disposal system of the cell.

mass synergies of movement   mass or gross movement patterns characterized by flexion in all joints of the limb or extension in all joints of the limb. These mass synergies characterize the basic spinal programmes of movement and are also seen in patients who have lost the ability to modify basic spinal activity.

mechanoceptor   the second part of the word *ceptor* refers to the transducer component of a sensory nerve ending. The first part of the word refers to the form of energy transduced, or changed in form. A *mechano*ceptor transduces the energy from a mechanical form to an electrical form capable of exciting the neuron terminal.

meiosis   (reduction division). Two successive divisions of a diploid cell. The number of chromosomes present in each of the daughter cells is half that of a diploid (q.v.) cell.

medial geniculate nucleus   a swelling on the ventral surface of the thalamus, forming part of the auditory pathway linking the inferior colliculus to the transverse temporal gyri.

microfilaments   thin filaments of actin (q.v.) found as a lattice underneath the neurite (q.v.) membrane, and as parallel fibres near points where growth cones (q.v.) attach to the extracellular matrix or other cells. They are involved in guidance of the growth cone (q.v.).

microtubules   long chains of tubulin (q.v.) passing down the central core of a neurite (q.v.). Microtubules form the tracks along which molecules and organelles are transported from the cell body (axonal transport) where they are made to the nerve endings where they are used.

mitochondria   intracellular organelles with double membranes. They are the site where energy from food (substrate molecules) is stored in adenosine triphosphate (q.v. ATP).

mitosis   the usual process by which a cell nucleus divides into two daughter cells. Each daughter cell has a full complement of chromosomes.

modality   the quality of sensory information, such as visual or auditory.

monomer   a molecular component being a single member of a process of polymerization (q.v.) where many monomers are bonded together. A dimer is two of the bonded components.

movement patterns, abnormal   movement patterns not normally seen in an adult. May consist of mass synergies of movement of the type produced by the isolated spinal cord.

movement patterns, fractionated movement patterns characterized by flexion in one joint and extension in another joint or an isolated movement in one joint only. They are a modification of basic spinal movements.

myofilament an individual skeletal muscle cell (or more exactly a syncytium of muscle cells) is called a muscle fibre and is approximately 100 μm in diameter. Each striated cell is composed of bundles of myofilaments. Each discrete bundle is referred to as myofibril.

NCAM an acronym for neuron, cell adhesion molecule. A membrane macromolecule important in neuron–neuron recognition and adhesion. A component molecule of the growth cone membrane (q.v.).

N-cadherin a cell adhesion molecule that depends on Ca^{2+} for its binding properties. It is found on the surface of neurons and contributes to the binding of one cell to another.

nerve cell adhesion molecule a cell adhesion molecule that acts independently of Ca^{2+}, found in nerve cell membranes. It contributes to the binding of one cell to another.

nerve growth factors an extracellular soluble protein necessary for the continued existence of dependent cells such as sympathetic neurons.

neurite a process of a neuron, either in the sense of primitive, e.g. invertebrate, or of immature in mammal, including humans. A developing or rehabilitating process. The site of the growth cone (q.v.).

neuroepithelial cells the sheet of embryonic cells from which the central nervous system is derived.

neurofilaments thin filaments found in the mature axons of neurons, aiding microtubules in axonal transport and providing a cross-linked scaffold that confers strength to the neurite (q.v.).

neurocrine a neuronal system which releases molecular signals to diffuse to closely adjacent target cells. A somewhat more diffuse system than the synaptic system. cf. endocrine and paracrine.

neuropil the axon terminals and dendrites that fill the space between cell bodies in the grey matter of the central nervous system.

neurotropic guiding the direction of growth of a neuron.

neurotrophic capable of supporting the continued existence of a neuron.

NgCAM an acronym for neuron–glia cell adhesion molecule. A component molecule of the growth cone membrane (q.v.).

NGF acronym for nerve growth factor. A molecule capable of steering the developing neurite (q.v.).

nigrostriatal tracts dopaminergic fibres passing from the substantia nigra to the corpus striatum, involved in Parkinson's syndrome.

Nissl substance the visible aspect of the RNA bound to granular endoplasmic reticulum. The protein synthesizing apparatus of the cell.

NMDA acronym for N-methyl D-aspartate. A receptor channel associated with Ca^{2+}. It acts as a ligand-gated channel (q.v.).

N-methyl D-aspartate receptor a Ca^{2+} channel opened by the binding of glutamate but blocked by Mg^{2+} unless there is sufficient depolarization to displace the cation from its orifice. Crucial in learning and development.

NPF acronym for neurite-promoting factor (q.v.). An important agent in neurogenesis.

ontogenetic the whole course of development of organs and systems during an individual's life history.

paracrine a system which releases molecular signals which influence target cells situated in close locality and in the same body fluid compartment. cf. endocrine and neurocrine.

passive stretch responses excessive EMG activity occurring in a muscle as a result of passive stretch. A characteristic of spasticity..

PET scans positron emission tomography scans. They detect the location of radioactive isotopes in the brain and can indicate which parts of it are metabolically active during a given activity.

phenotype the sum of characteristics manifested by an organism or a cell as contrasted with the set of genes possessed by it (q.v. genotype). The actuality of a cell compared with its potentiality.

phosphatidyl inositol biphosphate a fat soluble molecule that can be split by phospholipase C to give diacyl glycerol (q.v.) and inositol triphosphate (q.v.), both of which are important in cell signalling mechanisms. cf. second messengers.

phospholipase C an enzyme activated by G-protein (q.v.) and capable of splitting phosphatidyl inositol biphosphate into its components.

phosphorylation the addition of a phosphate group to a molecule, catalysed by an enzyme called a kinase. This is particularly important in activating or inactivating proteins.

phylogenetic a relationship based on closeness of evolutionary descent. (q.v. recapitulation).

polymer a compound formed by polymerization believed originally to be a chemical union of the same compound to form larger molecules of the same empirical formula. Biochemistry has extended this definition.

post-tetanic potentiation a short-lasting increase in the amplitude of postsynaptic potentials produced by high-frequency stimulation of the synapse.

postcentral gyrus the gyrus posterior to the central sulcus. It contains sensory representation of the skin and joints, but is now known to evoke movements that are linked to sensation. q.v. cortex, motosensory.

probability the likelihood of an event occurring, measured by the ratio of favourable cases to the whole number of cases possible. If an event can happen in a ways and fail in b ways, the probability of it happening is $a/(a +b)$.

proteoglycans   complex compounds made from protein and special carbohydrates called glycosaminoglycans.

protein kinase C   a protein that phosphorylates other proteins such as GAP43 (q.v.).

proto-oncogenes   genes whose products are growth factors, growth factor receptors or proteins that regulate with cell adhesion or the expression of other genes. They are the normal counterpart of viral genes that can induce the growth of tumours.

Purkinje cells   the final output cell of the cerebellar cortex. cf. hot spot.

projection fibres   cerebral cortical axons that link the cortex to subcortical structures.

quisqualate receptor   a receptor that binds glutamate and permits the entry of Na^+ into the cell.

radial glia   glial cells with long processes that extend from the subventricular zone to the cerebrocortical surface. Migrating neurons attach themselves to the radial glia.

recapitulation   occurrence in an individual during embryonic development, tissue repair and rehabilitation of a repetition of successively later embryonic stages corresponding to more recent ancestors. Ontogeny repeats phylogeny (q.v.)

rehabilitation   following damage to the central nervous system in adults restores to them, ideally, their previous function, usually their motor function.

reactive synaptogenesis   replacement of degenerated synapses by new synapses from axons in the vicinity of those that have been lost.

regulatory proteins   proteins that can enter a cell's nucleus and control the expression of its genes.

resting   potential. In the context of this book it means unexcited.

retrograde degeneration   degeneration of a neuron soma (cell body) as a result of destruction of its axon.

retrograde transport   the transport of material from the peripheral end of a neurite (q.v.) back to the soma (cell body).

ribosome   protein and RNA present in a free form in the cytoplasm as either a single molecular complex or in a cluster of such forms: the polyribosome. In a membrane bound form they are aligned along an extent of the endoplasmic reticulum. This intracellular canal system is given a rough appearance because of the granular ribosomes it is carrying. It is then known as the 'rough endoplasmic reticulum'.

RNA, messenger RNA, mRNA   ribonucleic acid molecule that conveys from chromosomal DNA the information needed for translation (q.v.) to a polypeptide chain.

RNA, ribosomal RNA, rRNA   one of the structural components of the ribosome (q.v.). Contributes to the capacity of the ribosome to attract and properly orient mRNA and tRNA.

RNA, transfer RNA, tRNA   a molecule responsible for recognizing and carrying an amino acid for translation (q.v.) into a polypeptide chain in response to information carried by mRNA and through the agency of a ribosome (q.v.).

rubrospinal tract   axons projecting from the red nucleus (n. ruber) to the spinal cord, thought to be involved in discrete movements of larger joints of the limbs.

sarcoplasmic reticulum   a tubular system in the cytoplasm (sarcoplasm) of striated muscle fibres. Responsible for sequestering free Ca^{2+} and holding it in bound form. Free Ca^{2+} is released by the action potential and acts as an electrical/mechanical link for muscle action.

saltatory   conduction in myelinated axons. From *saltum*, Latin: a leap. The electronic spread of electrical current through a neuron by cable conduction is a passive event and does not involve the molecules of the membrane other than as components of a physical conductor. But, if the passive current flow involves a patch of membrane as a 'hot-spot' (q.v.) or at a node of Ranvier an action potential is generated. This potential is localized to the patch of membrane where it was generated, but the passive flow of electrical currents it generates spreads by cable conduction and involves a 'hot-spot' or regenerative zone several millimetres away where a new action potential is generated. The action potential appears to leap in this way from node to node, and that mode of propagation is said to be saltatory. Propagation of action potentials in this way is rapid and efficient.

second messenger   a molecule or ion acting to transmit information during procedures of plastic adaptation. The first messenger is the neurotransmitter or hormone molecule and the third transmitter is the next molecule in a chain of instruction. A fourth messenger has been postulated.

sets, synaptic   an alternative way of classifying functional groups of neurons. A set of neurons can occupy any region of the central nervous system (CNS). The volume of CNS occupied may be defined in terms of the principal or projection neurons which are the only neurons whose axons leave the set. Intrinsic neurons of the set have axons which do not leave the set, but the extent of which again determines the volume of the set. Neurons afferent to the set, from central structures and from the periphery, have cell bodies outside the set, but axon terminals within it. A motor neuron pool of the spinal cord is an example of a set. A set may be formed during plastic adaptation through the influence of synaptic strength(ening) (q.v.).

smooth endoplasmic reticulum   a tubular network of membranes in the cytoplasm capable of sequestering Ca^{2+}. It is mainly responsible for part of fat metabolism. cf. sarcoplasmic reticulum.

soma   cell body of a neuron. The region of the neuron that contains the cell nucleus. The site of protein synthesis to the pattern instructed by genes and under the direction of messenger RNA (mRNA).

somatosensory cortex the postcentral gyrus, containing a sensory representation of skin and joints.

spines small projections of dendrites on which afferent terminals synapse. The number of spines formed is related to the activity in which the neurons are involved. In patients suffering sensory deprivation or mental retardation, the spines are sparse.

stochastic a numerical process which has some element of probability in its structure.

subventricular zone the layer outside the ependyma lining the cerebral ventricles, where the cell division giving rise to neurons takes place.

synaptic strength a way of expressing the amplitude of excitatory and inhibitory postsynaptic potentials (EPSP, IPSP). These local, non-propagated potentials depend upon the amount of neurotransmitter molecules stored in and released from the vesicles of the presynaptic ending, and the number of molecular receptor molecules found in the postsynaptic membrane. These factors and the transmitter-activated ion channels of the postsynaptic neuron are accessible to plastic adaptation.

talin one of the proteins that link actin to points of cellular attachment to the extracellular matrix.

tau protein a group of proteins associated with microtubules (q.v.), possibly involved in stabilizing them.

tissue culture growth of cells, including neurons, in an artificial medium. It is very useful for studying the behaviour of a small number of cell types under controlled conditions, but it is often very different from the real circumstances.

transcription synthesis of RNA, made up of a particular sequence of nucleotides, by matching with DNA, made up of a corresponding sequence of nucleotides.

translation synthesis of a polypeptide chain made up from a sequence of corresponding amino acids by matching with mRNA (q.v.) made up of a corresponding sequence of nucleotides.

transneural degeneration the degeneration of an uninjured neuron when the neuron with which it synapses has died.

tubulin the monomer (q.v.) from which microtubules (q.v.) are made.

vinculin one of the proteins that links actin (q.v.) to points of cell surface attachment.

voltage-gated channels ionophores (q.v.) that open or close in response to the prevailing potential difference across the cell membrane.

References

Abercrombie, M., Hickman, C. J. and Johnson, M. L. (1973) *A Dictionary of Biology*. London: The Penguin Group.

Reber, A. S. (1985) *Dictionary of Psychology*. London: The Penguin Group.

Index